Emerging Medical Technologies

Emerging Medical Technologies

Gennady Ermak
University of Southern California, USA

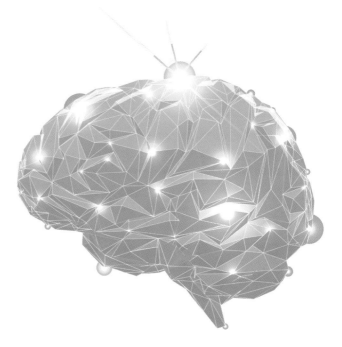

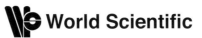

World Scientific

NEW JERSEY · LONDON · SINGAPORE · BEIJING · SHANGHAI · HONG KONG · TAIPEI · CHENNAI · TOKYO

Published by

World Scientific Publishing Co. Pte. Ltd.

5 Toh Tuck Link, Singapore 596224

USA office: 27 Warren Street, Suite 401-402, Hackensack, NJ 07601

UK office: 57 Shelton Street, Covent Garden, London WC2H 9HE

Library of Congress Cataloging-in-Publication Data
Ermak, Gennady.
   Emerging medical technologies / Gennady Ermak, University of Southern California, USA.
   pages cm
   Includes bibliographical references and index.
   ISBN 978-9814675802 (hardcover : alk. paper) -- ISBN 9814675806 (hardcover : alk. paper) --
   ISBN 978-9814675819 (pbk. : alk. paper) -- ISBN 9814675814 (pbk. : alk. paper)
   1. Medical innovations--History. I. Title.
   RA418.5.M4E76 2015
   610.28--dc23
                              2015023629

British Library Cataloguing-in-Publication Data
A catalogue record for this book is available from the British Library.

Printed in Singapore by Mainland Press Pte Ltd.

Contents

Acknowledgments

I am grateful to my colleagues Dr. James Figge, Dr. Jenny Ngo and Professor Anatoly Zhitkovich for their edits and suggestions. I am also indebted to my friends Gary Reichard, Christopher Harris and Francisco Paranada for their invaluable comments on the draft of this book and for correcting mistakes. Last but not least, it is a pleasure to give my thanks to my friend Denis Battocchio, and to my daughter Masha Ermak, for help with the illustrations.

Introduction

This book is essentially a new edition of the previous book titled *Modern Science & Future Medicine*. The title has been changed to reflect the subject more precisely. As biomedical science develops very fast, the current book has been updated with new information. Also, some mistakes made in the previous version have now been corrected.

This book is written for those who would like to understand the science behind modern and future medicine. It is written in a simple way that is understandable to the general public. Thus, it can be very useful for non-specialists that would like to catch up with quickly developing medical science. It is also a good starting point for students studying medicine/biology, as well as for professionals and specialists.

Medical technology is developing at the fastest pace ever. Many new drugs and treatments which improve the quality of medical care are becoming available every year. The media talks about this revolution in biology and medicine. Such rumors have already been going on for a few decades. Readers that went to school in the 1970s, 1980s, and 1990s are well aware of this! However, instead of this medical breakthrough, revolutions that nobody could have predicted came to pass: Cellular phones and the internet have revolutionized communications, as well as the media. So, what about the long-promised revolution in biology and medicine — is it really coming?

Although the talk has been going on for several decades, there has never been so much dramatic progress in medical science, all coming out at the same time, as there is now. New technologies, such as stem cell technology, pharmacogenomics (also called pharmacogenetics) and nano-technology, have the potential to revolutionize medicine. In addition, older technologies, such as gene therapy, genetic engineering, and cloning, are still in the first stages of development, and still hold great potential.

The book provides a comprehensive overview of the most important medicine-related technologies (most of which are familiar to everyone through the media): nanomedicine, cloning, stem cell technology, phar-macogenomics, gene therapy, and genetic engineering. An effort has been made to provide a minimal, yet sufficient scientific background, using graphics and diagrams to explain the basics of each technology in a simple manner. The description of each technology is structured in the same uni-fied way, and contains the following sub-topics: definition, history, prin-ciples, technical problems, past/present/future applications, controversies, and future. After reviewing and digesting the information provided, the reader will emerge with a general understanding of the science underlying modern medicine. Each chapter covers one of the medicine-related tech-nologies as follows:

1. Gene Therapy — This chapter defines gene therapy and distinguishes it from genetic engineering. It explains what genetic disorders are and discusses how gene therapy technology can correct them.

2. Genetic Engineering — This chapter provides examples of how this technology can be used by the pharmaceutical industry to produce a number of drugs. Since only part of this technology is directly applied to medicine, this chapter is brief.

3. Cloning — This chapter explains the difference between reproductive and therapeutic cloning. It analyzes the possible applications and limita-tions of this technology in manipulations with humans. In particular, the application of cloning to advance stem cell technology is discussed.

4. Stem Cells — This chapter explains what adult stem cells and what embryonic stem (ES) cells are. It explains how they can be developed, and discusses the currently existing controversies associated with stem cell research. This chapter also explains the advantages and disadvantages of one type of stem cell versus the other, and demonstrates that ES cells, which currently face so much controversy, might not even be necessary for future progress.

5. Nanomedicine — This chapter shows how this technology can revolutionize medical diagnostics and treatments. In particular, it describes how this technology can improve drug delivery systems, and its use in cancer treatments.

6. Pharmacogenomics — This chapter demonstrates how the genome of each individual is unique, and thus explains why some drugs might work for one patient, but not for another. It explains how doctors can now design drug treatments for each patient individually.

7. Other Technologies — This chapter briefly describes new scientific developments in the field of genetics, computer biology, and robotics that can further revolutionize medical technologies.

8. Modern Science and Dietary Supplements — Dietary supplements play an important role in modern life, and this book would not be complete without their consideration. The latest research demonstrates that supplements may cause more harm than good. This chapter discusses the health effects of supplements and explains why they can be dangerous for one's health.

Technological advances in modern medicine raise controversies and ignite public debates. For example, currently, there are debates over whether embryonic stem cell research should be allowed, or whether human cloning should even be permitted. Some people believe it should, while others are deeply opposed. As a result, some governments permit the research and development of these technologies, while others do not. In order for an informed opinion to be formed regarding the use of such technologies, one must understand their basics. However, most of these technologies are so new that most people could not possibly have learned about them at school. Conversely, there is a shortage of literature that covers them in a concise and simple way. This book is intended to address these shortcomings.

CHAPTER 1

Gene Therapy

Definition

Gene therapy is the treatment of disease by repairing or reconstructing defective genetic material. This technique was originally designed to correct human genetic disorders caused by abnormalities in the genetic material. Such disorders can be caused by abnormalities in a single gene (for the definition of "gene," see below), a combination of abnormalities in several genes, abnormalities in the chromosome structure, or mutations in the genetic material of mitochondria (cell organelles that produce energy). Current gene therapy technology focuses primarily on the correction of abnormalities caused by a single gene or by several genes. Therefore, modern gene therapy can be defined as a technique that replaces one (defective or undesirable) gene with another (normal or therapeutic) one. It is important to note that this technology is not intended to change the human genome (the collection of all genes), nor to introduce any non-human genes into human cells. This is what distinguishes gene therapy from genetic engineering, which is intended not just to repair an existing genome, but to create new genomes that do not exist in nature. Gene therapy has now been under development for several decades, but so far it has not produced any clear-cut therapeutic results, and it can still be considered to be in its infancy.

Each year, over 150,000 babies born in the US, and an estimated 3,000,000 babies worldwide, have birth defects. More than 6,000 single-gene disorders are currently known. Among the disorders are cystic fibrosis, sickle cell anemia, Huntington's disease, hemophilia, and others. Each and every person carries at least several defective genes. Fortunately, most of these defects are not life-threatening, and do not cause any obvious abnormalities. However, this has a down side: Defective genes that do not cause serious defects or death are easily transmitted from parents to children. Also, as humans learn how to treat genetic disorders, more and more people carrying defective genes survive and pass them through successive generations, leading to the gradual accumulation of gene defects in future generations. For example, the genetic defect that causes hemophilia: People with hemophilia lack a particular protein involved in blood clotting, and thus lack the ability to stop bleeding. Even minor injuries that are harmless to most people can be fatal to hemophiliacs. However, if hemophiliac patients receive appropriate care, they will survive and pass on the defective gene. A good illustration of this comes from the European royal families, in which the defective gene was easily passed from Queen Victoria to the royal families of Russia, Prussia, and Spain.

The human genome consists of 23 pairs of chromosomes (46 chromosomes total). One of the chromosomes from each pair originates from the mother, and the other one from the father. Thus, each gene is present in duplicate, or pairs (one copy from each parent). Very often however, one gene from a pair "contradicts" the instructions of the other. For example, one gene might instruct the eyes to be blue, while the other gene carries the instructions for brown eyes. In such situations, the body has to decide which gene controls eye color. The controlling gene is called the "dominant" gene, while the second (silent) one is called the "recessive" gene. In this particular case, the gene responsible for brown eyes is dominant, while the gene responsible for blue eyes is recessive. In some situations, a defect in a single dominant gene will cause a problem. On the other hand, if a single recessive gene is defective, it will be compensated for, if it is paired with a normally-functioning dominant gene, therefore preventing harm. However, if an individual is unfortunate enough to inherit a defective recessive gene from each parent, resulting in two recessive genes, then a disease can arise because there is no normal dominant gene to compensate the defective recessive gene.

The pair of sex chromosomes is an exception. Females have two X chromosomes (XX), while males have one X chromosome and one Y chromosome (XY). Thus, genes in the male pair of chromosomes are not duplicated, and defects in the X chromosome cannot be compensated by the Y chromosome, thereby causing so-called X-linked genetic diseases. Perhaps the best known example of such diseases is hemophilia. If a male inherits the defective X gene, he will always develop this disease, whereas both X genes must be defective to cause hemophilia in a female.

History

Gene therapy for human genetic diseases was first conceptualized in 1972.[1] Attempts to correct genes were soon made, but were not successful. An important step in the development of gene therapy technology is the delivery of therapeutic genes into human cells. Viruses can be easily used to transport therapeutic genes but, unfortunately, they normally cause diseases. Fortunately, a breakthrough came in 1984, when viruses were altered in such a way that they became safe for use in human gene therapy procedures.

The first gene therapy clinical trial was performed in 1990 in the US, when a patient was treated for ADA-SCID (for more, see Ref. 2). Over 1,000 other clinical trials were approved worldwide since then, most of them in the US.[3] Unfortunately, none of them have been considered completely successful to date. Even worse, several trials had to be stopped due to the danger of side effects, such as cancer and death. The first blow to this research came in 1999, when an 18-year old man died in the US in a trial targeting ornithine transcarbamylase deficiency (OTCD). He died from multiple organ failure just four days after the treatment, and it is believed that his death was triggered by a severe immune response to the adenoviral vectors (defined below) that were used to deliver the therapeutic gene. Another setback came from France in 2003. In this trial, 11 boys were treated using retroviral vectors for X-linked severe combined immunodeficiency (X-SCID). Two of them subsequently developed a leukemia-like condition, which was a side effect of the retroviral vectors.[4] Nevertheless, one can argue that this trial was not a failure, as is widely considered, but rather the first success. It seems that the other nine boys out of the total 11 are just fine, while the two boys that acquired the leukemia-like condition are undergoing treatment and may recover.

These side effects and failures prompted authorities around the world to take a fresh look at gene therapy trials and to put some of them on hold. As a result, the number of approved gene therapy clinical trials declined from 116 in 1999 to just 73 in 2011.[3] Although this slowed down progress in western nations, it did not affect some others. In 2003, China's State Food and Drug Administration approved the first gene therapy product for clinical use in humans.[5] This product, Gendicine, is used against various forms of cancer (see more details in Applications). Also, the first such product has been finally approved in the West. The European Commission has recently given authorization to the small Dutch company, uniQure, to treat people with a rare genetic disorder, beginning of summer 2013 (see more details in Applications).

Principles

Gene therapy is done by replacement of a defective gene with a normal one. To deliver the genes into certain types of cells, and into the appropriate place inside of the cells, viruses and other carriers are used. Therefore, to understand how gene therapy works, one must first know what a gene is, and then how it can be transferred using viral and non-viral carriers.

(1) **Gene** — Genes are stored in DNA, a component of chromosomes, which are located in the nucleus of a cell. Some genes are also located in another cell compartment, called mitochondria. However, the main function of mitochondria is to produce energy for the cell. Also, human mitochondria have only 37 genes, as opposed to the approximately 30,000 genes contained in the nucleus.

DNA contains all of the instructions for cell functions. To "read" these instructions, pieces of DNA are first copied (transcribed); the copies, called RNAs, are then usually transported from the nucleus into the cytoplasm, where they instruct the cell to produce proteins, which serve as the functional building blocks of the body. Traditionally, a piece of DNA that encodes a protein was called a gene. Recently, however, this definition has expanded to include segments of DNA that encode RNAs, because not all RNAs carry the instructions to build proteins. Some RNAs are used to produce proteins and other RNAs serve as the regulators. Currently, the most acceptable definition of a gene is: a DNA sequence that encodes an RNA molecule. However, the discussion over the definition of "gene" will continue to evolve as more is learned.

The collection of all genes from one single cell is called a genome. With few exceptions, genomes of cells originating from the same organism are identical, no matter from which organ or tissue. Let us take, for example, your own body: Genomes of neuronal and muscle (or any other) cells taken from your body will be 100% identical, despite the fact that these cells look completely different. One notable exception is certain cells comprising the immune system, where the DNA rearrangements occur in different patterns in different immune cells. This mechanism allows immune cells to recognize a large variety of foreign substances. On the other hand, the genome from your neuronal cell and the genome from the neuronal cell of any other person (except in case of identical twins) will be slightly different, even if the cells appear identical. The slight differences in the genome from one person to the next are responsible for the unique characteristics of each individual. Nevertheless, all human genomes are at least 99% alike.

How does it happen that nearly all cells in the same body have the same genes, but they look different, and they do different jobs? This is because only certain groups of genes are active in any cell at any given moment, while the rest of the genes are "silent." As cells develop and grow, different genes become active or inactive. Actually, it would be correct to say that gene activation and inactivation prompt cells to develop, grow, or to do whatever else. The set of active and inactive genes in cells determines both how they look and what they do.

The human genome contains about 30,000 genes. The genome is stored in the cell nucleus, which can be easily seen under a light microscope. Nuclei contain smaller structures, called chromosomes. Chromosomes are composed of DNA as well as proteins, and proteins have a supportive function in chromosomes. In turn, the DNA is composed of four chemicals that are called nucleotides (A, T, G, and C), much like a four-letter alphabet. These four chemicals bind to each other in a specific order to form the sequence of the DNA, for example

...ATTTTCCG... and so on. Each DNA strand consists of more than one billion nucleotides, strung together in a precise linear sequence. Amazingly, the linear order of just these four chemicals encodes the blue-print of our life — it determines the color of our eyes, it controls how tall we can grow, and what diseases we are prone to.

(A) *How genes work*: A gene is a piece of DNA that tells cells how to do a particular job. Genes instruct cells on how to build RNAs and pro-teins, and when to start or stop such production. Proteins are not manu-factured in the nucleus, where genes are located, but rather in the cytoplasm. Genes send instructions from the nucleus to the cytoplasm using molecules called RNAs (see Fig. 1.1). Pieces of DNA, called genes, are copied in the nucleus (this process is called transcription). The copies, called messenger RNAs, are then transported into the cytoplasm, where they are used as instructions to build proteins (this process is called transla-tion). Proteins are built from chemicals called amino acids. The nucleotide sequence of an RNA determines the amino acid sequence of the corre-sponding protein. Specifically, each consecutive group of three nucleotides of RNA provides the code for an amino acid that will be used next to build a protein. For example, the AAG nucleotide sequence instructs that the amino acid lysine should be used to build a protein, while the AGG sequence will instruct that the amino acid arginine should be used.

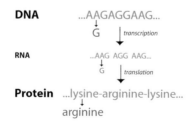

Fig. 1.1   Genes instruct the synthesis of proteins. In this particular example, the gene sequence ...AAGAGGAAG... instructs that the sequence of a synthesized protein should be lysine-arginine-lysine. Any single mistake in the gene sequence can lead to the synthesis of a protein that has the wrong sequence. For example, the exchange of the second nucleotide A for G will lead to the synthesis of a protein in which the amino acid lysine is replaced by the amino acid arginine, which consequently might cause a protein to function abnormally or not to function at all.

The vast majority of DNA (about 97%) contained in human chromosomes does not make up genes. The role of this non-genic DNA is not yet understood. This DNA might regulate the expression of genes. It might also represent old ancestor genes, as well as new evolving genes, and it might be necessary for gene evolution. Most research is currently devoted to genes only, without serious consideration for the remaining more than 90% of DNA. Step by step, genes are sequenced, and we learn how they work. But even if one discovers them all, science might still be far from understanding exactly how the human genome works, because we know almost nothing about the rest of the DNA.

(B) *How to make genes*: In order to synthesize a gene, we need to know its DNA sequence. In other words, the gene must first be decoded. Based on the sequence, we can make genes in several ways. The first step, however, is always the same — DNA that contains genes must be isolated from cells, and then purified. Then, DNA fragments representing the gene of interest either can be "cut out" of the total DNA using special enzymes, or they can be synthesized by a technique called "polymerase chain reaction" (PCR).

(C) *Where to deliver*: Depending on the goals of the therapy, genes can be transferred either into germ (egg or sperm) cells or into somatic cells (any other cells in our bodies). When genes are transferred into someone's germ cells, they can be passed on to the offspring, while genes transferred into somatic cells cannot be passed on. The germ-line gene transfer is widely used for manipulations with animals, but not with humans, because of technical and ethical issues. Most of the current human gene therapy trials are performed using somatic cells, as shown in Fig. 1.2.

(D) *How to deliver*: Delivery of therapeutic genes into cells is not an easy task. Cells are covered with membranes that isolate them from the environment, and allow only select molecules to penetrate. Membranes do not let manufactured or foreign DNA fragments (representing laboratory isolated genes) to penetrate cells. Therefore, genes must be forcefully delivered across membranes, and several methods currently exist to do this. One way is to isolate a fragment of DNA containing the desirable genes, then break the membrane, and allow the genes to freely flow inside

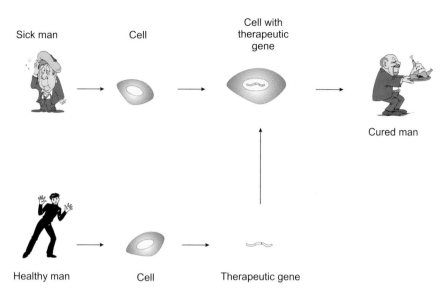

Fig. 1.2   Principles of somatic cell gene therapy. To correct a defective gene, cells are isolated from a sick patient who has the defective gene, and the normally functioning gene isolated from a healthy man is then delivered into these cells. The cells with the new normal gene are then transplanted back into the sick patient, where they divide and replace cells with the defective gene, curing the patient.

the cells, hoping that they will eventually integrate into the host DNA and repair the defective genome. Another method involves special delivery molecules called "vectors." In this case, DNA with a desirable gene is first inserted into the vector, and then the vector delivers the gene into cells. Currently, the most popular vectors are viruses. However, viruses can transfer only relatively small DNA fragments, and scientists are working to develop artificial chromosomes that can be used as vectors, in order to operate with larger DNA fragments.

(2) **Viral Gene Delivery** — DNA or RNA, which contains genetic information, is the main component of viruses. Viruses "know" how to exploit human cells. They penetrate into human cells, integrate their genetic information into the host genome, and use the cells to reproduce themselves. Humans are now learning how to exploit viruses. Scientists can now isolate therapeutic human genes and insert them into the viral genome while taking the toxic viral genes out of the viral genome. These

"disarmed" viruses then can infect human cells and deliver the desirable genes into the human genome without actually causing disease. Several types of viruses are currently used as vectors:

(A) *Adenoviruses*: These are common human viruses that cause respiratory, intestinal, and eye infections. For example, the common cold virus is an adenovirus. The main part of adenoviruses is composed of double-stranded DNA. These viruses infect many types of human cells, and are currently the most commonly used vectors in gene therapy clinical trials. About 23% of all trials by the year 2011 made use of this method of gene delivery.[3]

(B) *Retroviruses*: A well-known example of this type of virus is HIV. However, the less-known Moloney murine leukemia virus, rather than HIV, is used to create retroviral vectors. Retroviruses have RNA instead of DNA. After infection, however, this RNA is converted into double-stranded DNA, which then integrates into the human genome. Since retroviruses infect various cell types, they can be used to deliver therapeutic genes into many tissues and organs. Retroviruses are the second most commonly used vectors after adenoviruses, and by the year 2005 about 20% of all clinical trials used retroviral methods of gene delivery.[3]

(C) *Herpes simplex viruses.* These are common human pathogens that cause cold sores (herpes). These viruses contain double-stranded DNA, which infects mainly one type of human cell: neurons. Thus, these vectors are good candidates to repair defective genes in the brain and nervous system.

(D) *Adeno-associated viruses.* These viruses are composed of single-stranded DNA molecules, and can infect several types of cells. Unlike other viruses, which randomly insert their genetic material into the host genome, these viruses always insert their genes into a specific site of the human genome, which is located on chromosome 19. Because of this, they allow for the insertion of trans-genes in a predictable manner, and are gaining popularity in gene therapy. Moreover, these vectors have been shown to even cross the blood–brain barrier,[6] which could eliminate the need for difficult medical procedures, such as skull-drilling, to deliver vectors into the brain.

(3) **Non-Viral Gene Delivery** — There are several techniques to deliver genes into cells without viral vectors. A simple way is to make holes in the

membrane through which DNA fragments can freely flow into the cell before the membrane is repaired. Holes can be produced by the use of an electric shock, among other techniques. These techniques, however, have a significant drawback: The cells become stressed and damaged.

Another, gentler way, is to pack genes into liposomes. Liposomes are artificial lipid spheres with an aqueous core, in which DNA can be dissolved. These lipid spheres packed with DNA can easily pass across the cell membrane, delivering therapeutic genes inside cells. Instead of packing genes into liposomes, DNA can also be chemically bound to special molecules that bind to membrane receptors. After the binding, they can be engulfed by the membrane, transporting genes into the cell interior. This delivery system, however, is not very efficient.

Finally, genes can be transferred into cells simply by injection, using fine glass needles. This method is called pronuclear injection, and it allows passing not only the cell membrane but also the nuclear membrane, thus delivering genes directly into the nuclei, the cell compartments where DNA is stored. It is mostly used to deliver genes into germ cells (such as eggs). The disadvantage of this method is that it is stressful for cells and it is labor-intensive.

Technical Problems

Gene therapy has shown itself to not be as simple as originally contemplated. Many problems have to be solved before it becomes an effective treatment:

(1) **Delivering Genes to the Right Place** — Non-viral gene therapy techniques allow genes to be either delivered directly into the cytoplasm (from where it needs to penetrate into nuclei) or directly into the nuclei. What happens next is that DNA fragments, which carry therapeutic genes (transgenes), just flow around the host DNA and are randomly inserted into the genome by a process called recombination. And this randomness is a problem. In order to function properly, genes have to be delivered to the right place. If a trans-gene is inserted into a random host gene, it will disrupt, inactivate, or transform it. Depending on which host gene is affected, this

can result in various diseases, or have little effect. Even if it is not inserted into the host gene, but rather, into the non-coding DNA strand between two host genes, it can still cause a problem. For example, the non-coding DNA might be at the site that regulates the expression of genes. Thus, disruption of this DNA region could lead to the unnatural induction or the inhibition of host genes. Once again, depending on which genes are affected, it might lead to various diseases, including cancer.

If viruses are used for gene delivery, the results are similar. Most viruses infect cells and insert their genes into the host DNA in a random fashion, which causes the same problems. The major exceptions are the adeno-associated viruses, which insert their genetic material into a specific site, that of chromosome 19.

(2) **Delivering Intact Genes** — As therapeutic genes are transferred, they might be partially deleted or mutated before they become functional. This may disable or silence the therapeutic gene. On the other hand, there is a chance that altered therapeutic genes can still be expressed, producing a wrong and harmful result.

(3) **Inserting the Right Number of Therapeutic Genes** — Another problem of both viral and non-viral delivery techniques is our inability to control the number of therapeutic genes transferred into one cell. As most current techniques generally require millions of copies of a therapeutic gene per one cell, with the hopes that at least one copy will be successfully integrated, an unlimited number of copies can be inserted into the cell. This might cause not only alterations and rearrangements of host genes, but also excessive levels of the trans-gene production, if more than one copy is inserted.

(4) **Making Trans-Genes Long-Lived** — In order to achieve sustained success, therapeutic genes must be functional for the lifetime of the patient. When viruses are used to express a therapeutic gene, problems can arise due to the fact that the reproduction rates of viruses fluctuate and generally decrease after transfer, which leads to the decreased production of therapeutic genes. However, if the trans-gene is inserted into the host genome, it does not need the virus for expression. Unfortunately, most cells undergoing gene therapy constantly divide and, for whatever

reason, they either lose trans-genes or gradually lower their expression. This problem can be corrected through repeated therapy. This, of course, increases the cost of therapy, and makes it inconvenient for patients. Even more importantly, it increases chances of the elimination of the trans-genes by the immune system, which "sees" them as foreign objects (please see explanations below).

(5) **The Immune Rejection** — The immune system normally recognizes foreign entities and eliminates them from our bodies. This protects us from infections and helps us fight diseases. When therapeutic genes are delivered using vectors (for example, viruses), the immune system "does not understand" that this is actually something good for our body, and fights back, eliminating the vectors and trans-genes altogether. Even if gene therapy is performed using no vectors, it can still cause an immune response due to the fact that, most of time, trans-genes are inappropriately inserted into the host genome. Such inappropriate insertion then causes altered gene expression in the treated cells, which makes them look like foreign objects and targets for elimination by the immune system.

(6) **Fluctuating Levels of the Host Gene Expression** — In current gene therapy techniques, the therapeutic gene is always "on," working and producing proteins constantly. Normal cells, however, express some genes only at certain developmental stages, whose expression at other stages can be harmful. Therefore, the regulation of trans-gene expression systems is necessary in order to more efficiently repair these types of genes, and such systems are in need of further development.

Applications

Numerous trials, intended to correct various diseases using gene therapy, are currently under way. They include trials of vascular and infectious diseases, among others. But most of them (about 67% of all gene therapy trials) address cancer.

(1) **ADA Deficiency** — ADA deficiency was the first disease approved for gene therapy treatment. The reason it has been chosen is that this disease is relatively well understood. It is caused by the abnormality of one single

gene that produces an enzyme called adenosine deaminase (ADA). Thus, correction of just this one gene will treat the disease. A defect of this gene causes some form of Severe Combined Immunodeficiency (SCID). More exactly, ADA deficiency makes up about 20% of all SCID cases. As the name suggests, SCID causes deficiencies in the immune system. Children born with this defect become highly susceptible to infections. If untreated, ADA is lethal, and can cause death from infections within six months of birth. The exact mechanism of how the defect in the ADA gene causes the disease is unknown. However, it can be treated by the intravenous injection of the drug called PEG-ADA, which is essentially the same protein produced by a normal ADA gene. The problem is that this treatment, by injection, has to continue for one's whole life, and it costs about $100,000 per year, while the gene therapy approach promises to correct the problem once and for all, for the rest of the patient's life.

The most popular approach for the treatment of SCID was to use retroviral vectors. Viral vectors, however, have a number of problems, as described previously, and despite the relative simplicity, so far, ADA deficiency has not been successfully treated. Approaches to treat ADA that combine gene therapy with new technologies, such as stem cell technology, are currently underway. Some success has also been achieved using umbilical cord blood cells, and it is possible that this disease will become curable within the next several years. In fact, it has been recognized that in the last decade, gene therapy has been developed as the most successful and safest alternative strategy for patients affected by ADA-SCID.[7]

(2) **Sickle Cell Disease** — It was widely believed that this disease would be the first genetic disorder treated using gene therapy. But the task proved to be far more challenging than originally thought, and since the first experiments in 1979, the struggle to cure it still continues. The disease is caused by a mutation in a single gene that encodes the oxygen-transporting protein in blood, called beta-globin. The mutation leads to an abnormal shape of red blood cells, and thus renders them ineffective. Red blood cells are produced in the bone marrow from progenitor stem cells. Therefore, if the gene in those few stem cells can be fixed (as shown in Fig. 1.2), the disorder can be cured. However, delivering the gene into the correct place in the host genome, which would allow the gene to

express itself at the right levels and for a lifetime, is the main obstacle in these trials. Definite success has currently been achieved using animal models, in which the gene therapy resulted in full restoration of red blood cells for a significantly long period. However, several safety issues still must be resolved before the procedure can be applied to humans.

(3) **X-Linked Severe Combined Immunodeficiency (X-SCID)** — This is also known as "baby in the bubble" disease. It seems that this disorder may be the first disease treated successfully using gene therapy. Similarly to the above-described ADA deficiency, X-SCID causes another form of SCID. In fact, it is the most common form of SCID, and includes 46–70% of all SCID cases, affecting at least 1 in 100,000 births. It has an "X" in the name because the gene responsible for the disease, called the IL2RG gene, is located on the X-chromosome. This gene encodes the protein that is important for the growth and activation of the immune system. Mutations in this gene lead to a number of pathologies, including immuno-deficiencies that can be life-threatening. If untreated, newborn babies usually do not survive past infancy. In females, this mutated gene is usually compensated for by the normal IL2RG gene on the second X-chromosome, rendering them unsusceptible to the disease. Males, however, have only one X-chromosome. Thus, the abnormal gene cannot be compensated for, and when the IL2RG gene is mutated, the disease always manifests.

X-SCID can be treated in babies by bone marrow transplantation, using bone marrow from another individual with the normal gene. Nevertheless, this operation is complex, and only partially restores function. Patients who receive transplants do not always achieve full immune recovery, and may still suffer from infections and other problems. Thus, further improvements in this disease treatment are still a pressing matter, and gene therapy looks to be the most promising answer. In 2000, a team in France pioneered this treatment and replaced the faulty IL2RG gene, using a retroviral vector gene delivery system. At first, the procedure seemed like a complete success and a miracle. Later, however, two out of the 11 boys enrolled in the trial developed a leukemia-like condition, which was due to the insertion of the retrovirus at an inappropriate location in the genome of these two boys. Specifically, the virus was inserted into the DNA region that controls LMO2 proto-oncogene (the gene that can transform normal cells into cancerous cells), which led to the over-production of immune cells in the blood. This raised questions about the safety of the procedure, and led to the temporary suspension of such trials around the world. Nevertheless, this trial can be considered a success: The other patients are doing well, and for some of them, the procedure was indeed a miracle. It is also worth noting that some children with X-SCID cannot be helped with the current treatments, using bone marrow transplants, and will die. Thus, gene therapy is the only chance for survival, and a step worth taking for these children. For this reason, X-SCID trials were not suspended in some countries. For example, a trial involving seven children was allowed to continue in the UK.[8] Scientists are now adjusting procedures to avoid interference of trans-genes with host genes, and these trials are slowly starting to resume. Current common consensus is that the past 20 years have shown that X-SCID conditions are correctable through gene therapy.[9]

(4) **Leber's Congenital Amaurosis (LCA)** — LCA is a rare, inherited retinal disorder that causes blindness. It is caused by a defect in the RPE65 gene. In 2008, one group from the UK and two groups from the US independently reported successful replacement of the defective RPE65 gene with a functional copy, using adeno-associated viral vectors. Patients' vision was restored without apparent side-effects in all three trials, and this success provided much-needed optimism necessary for further investments in gene therapy.

(5) **Acquired Immune Deficiency Syndrome (AIDS)** — AIDS is caused by infection from the human immunodeficiency virus (HIV). Currently, there are many drugs that can be used to suppress HIV in the human body and slow down the progression of AIDS development. Unfortunately, these drugs only control, but do not cure, the disease. They are not capable of eradicating the virus from the body, and if not administered, HIV multiplies again and can lead to AIDS. A glimpse of hope in curing the disease came from Germany, when a patient was cured using a gene therapy approach. In this approach, the patient's normal CCR5 gene was replaced with a mutated one. HIV uses the host CCR5 protein to attach to the host immune cells and infect them. When this

protein is mutated, HIV cannot attach anymore, and patients become resistant to the virus. Thus, in 2007, researchers ablated bone marrow cells carrying the normal CCR5 gene in an HIV-infected patient (bone marrow contains stem cells that give rise to immune cells). Then, they replaced the normal CCR5 gene in stem cells with the mutated gene, and transplanted the cells into the HIV patient. He became completely resistant to HIV infections and thus cured (full story in Ref. 10). Although this approach is not yet accepted as a cure against HIV/AIDS, due to the difficulties of bone marrow replacement, it demonstrates that a cure is possible. Similar approaches are now being tested by researchers at the University of California in Los Angeles, in the US, with the hope of developing acceptable procedures for curing HIV/AIDS.

(6) **Cancers** — All cancers arise as the result of uncontrolled cell division. However, they are caused by a number of factors, and many genes are involved in tumorigenesis. Some genes (oncogenes) can induce uncontrolled cell division, and deleting or turning them "off" can prevent cancers. In contrast, other genes (tumor suppressor genes) serve to control cell division, and "implanting" them into cells or turning them "on" can be used to fight cancers. This principle was used to create the first-ever gene therapy product for clinical use in humans. As mentioned above, in 2003, the Chinese State Food and Drug Administration approved Gendicine.[5] This product represents a recombinant adenovirus, carrying a normal copy of the tumor suppressor gene, *p53*. It is designed to treat patients with the mutated *p53* gene, and is used against head/neck carcinoma and other cancer types. In China, this treatment is available at the relatively modest price of about $20,000 per two-month course.

The immune system recognizes and kills cancerous cells, and weakening of the immune system increases the chance of cancer growth. Therefore, the other currently used way to fight cancers employs the introduction or activation of genes that stimulate the patient's immune response against cancers.

As cancer grows, it needs more and more blood supply, which is facilitated by the growth of new blood vessels (this process is called angiogenesis). Thus, cancers can also be fought by manipulating genes that prevent angiogenesis.

Approaches involving genes that do not naturally regulate cancer development are also currently used. For example, researchers identified several genes that command cells to commit suicide (this process is called apoptosis). Induction of these "suicidal" genes within cancer cells can help to get rid of the cancer.

Widely used methods to kill cancer cells in clinics are chemotherapy (treatment with drugs) and radiotherapy (treatment with radiation). The expression of several genes was found to increase sensitivity of cells to these therapies. Thus, manipulating these genes can be used to increase the efficiency of both chemo- and radiotherapy.

Some cancers can also arise as a result of defects in a single gene. The treatment of such cancers using gene therapy is feasible in the near future, as compared to most cancers, whose nature is complex or not yet understood. Great resources have been deployed in this field; the majority of gene therapy clinical trials (about 67% in 2005) are targeted towards cancer treatment. Accordingly, it is reasonable to hope that at least a few of them (out of several hundred) will be successful, and that more gene therapy products will soon be used for cancer treatments.

(7) **Other Diseases** — Diseases that are caused by defects of one single gene are the easiest targets for gene therapy, and this procedure will have the greatest impact on the treatment of such diseases first. Among them are the above-described ADA deficiency, sickle cell disease, and X-SCID. Several other single gene disorders, such as hemophilia and phenylketonuria (PKU), are also the subject of current clinical trials, raising hopes that these diseases might also soon be successfully treated using gene therapy. Indeed, the world's second gene therapy product for clinical use, Glybera, is designed to treat people with a defect in the single gene that encodes lipoprotein lipase. Individuals with this defective gene are unable to break down fats, which leads to their build up, abdominal pain and life-threatening inflammation of the pancreas. Glybera represents a recombinant virus carrying a normal gene for the lipoprotein lipase. It works by infecting muscle cells with a normal copy of the gene and restoring the patient's ability to break down fats. This product is being developed by the Dutch company uniQure. It was approved in Europe in 2012 to become the first gene therapy drug of the Western world. However, its launch was delayed

in order to collect more data on its benefits. Soon, Glybera is set to go on scale in Germany at a staggering cost of €1.1 million ($1.4 million), which will make it the most expensive medicine in the world.

Most diseases, however, are caused by defects in several genes, as is in familial forms of Alzheimer's disease, and in most cancers. Using gene therapy for the treatment of these diseases is much more challenging, and probably will not occur within the next decade.

(8) **Unintended Applications** — Fantasies of possible gene therapy applications have played, and continue to play a role in popular culture. For example, gene therapy is the central element in the video game *Metal Gear Solid*, where it is used to enhance the fighting capabilities of soldiers. It was explored in the sci-fi television program *ReGenesis*, where it was used to enhance the performance of athletes. But are those ideas far from reality? Apparently not — gene therapy has already been used for illegal performance enhancement by athletes. Experiments with mice showed that gene therapy can dramatically boost their physical performance. In these experiments, mice were injected with a viral construct that carries the muscle-boosting gene IGF-1. Then, the endurance of the animals was tested by measuring how long they could swim before exhaustion. The doped mice swam three times as long, compared to the control group of animals (more details in Ref. 11).

Controversies

As with many new technologies, gene therapy raises some ethical and moral issues. At first, no clear distinction between gene therapy and genetic engineering was drawn, and many controversies associated with genetic engineering (which is the gene manipulation technology that aims to create organisms with unnatural properties, see Chapter 2) were auto-matically linked to gene therapy. Nevertheless, gene therapy in and of itself raises many controversies, and it is likely that they will become even stronger as the technology progresses and is used more frequently.

(1) **Harmfulness** — Harm can arise due to technical problems, as described above. For example, harmful consequences will arise if a

trans-gene is inserted in the wrong place in a host genome, or if several trans-genes are inserted into one cell, or if a disrupted trans-gene is inserted into cells. All of these events can cause harm and worsen a patient's condition. To deal with this issue, the potential risks of a therapy should be balanced against its potential benefits, and the therapy should only be used in cases in which the benefits clearly outweigh the risks. However, with progress, technical problems will gradually be solved, and as they are solved, this ethical issue will diminish in the future.

(2) **Inability to Consent** — This issue is associated with the germ-line gene therapy designed to correct germ cells from which a baby will originate. Such therapy is intended to prevent or alleviate disease before it happens. For example, if a mother carries mutated copies of the blood factor IX gene in both of her X-chromosomes, it means that if she gives birth to a boy, the boy will have hemophilia (please see explanations above). The disease could be prevented by gene therapy before this boy's birth. However, given that the boy is not yet born, he cannot consent to have his blood factor IX gene corrected. It is very unlikely that anybody would argue against the correction of his genes in this particular case, or in other cases when a gene defect is clearly life-threatening. Some genetic defects, however, are not such a clear threat, and decision-making in such cases may be challenging. To solve this issue, a list of diseases that are legitimate for germ-line therapy will eventually need to be developed and approved. Currently, however, there are no germ-line clinical trials underway, and this issue is not concern for now.

(3) **Fairness** — Genetic manipulation may potentially be used not just to treat a disease, but also to enhance or improve functions in normal people. For example, it can be used to help a person lose weight, grow taller, change eye color, enhance physical performance, or perhaps further in the future to enhance intelligence. Clearly, there will be a number of people willing to enhance one function or another, and it is unlikely that society will be able to afford this. This raises the questions: Who really needs this, and who will be the first? At the present, such gene corrections are not being developed, and do not really pose a problem. There is also consensus that genetic manipulations designed to enhance functions should not

be considered gene therapy, but rather as a part of genetic engineering, meaning this ethical issue is a problem associated with genetic engineering, rather than with gene therapy.

(4) **Assigning Biological Parents** — This ethical issue arises when mitochondrial genes are corrected. As we mentioned above, our genes are stored in chromosomes, which are located in cell nuclei. Several genes in human cells, however, are stored in mitochondria, which are located in the cytoplasm instead of the nucleus. Although there are only 37 genes in mitochondria (as compared to about 30,000 in nuclei), mitochondrial gene defects can cause serious problems. For example, they can cause infertility in women.

Most cells contain several/many mitochondria, except for sperm cells. Thus, mitochondrial genes originate only from eggs, and are inherited from a mother, but not from a father. To correct mitochondrial gene defects, specialists replace the whole cytoplasm containing all of the mitochondria, rather than correcting the defective gene in each mitochondrion. One way of doing this is to take the nucleus from an egg in which the mitochondria have genetic defects, and to place it into an egg containing normal mitochondria, but in which the original nucleus was removed (Fig. 1.3). This begs the question — where does the cell without the nucleus come from? It has to come from another woman. And this creates an ethical dilemma: Who should be considered the mother of the baby originating from such an egg? Now the baby has three parents — two women and one man. The current assumption is that the mother is the one from whom the nucleus was used to produce the baby. However, not everybody agrees.

Another way to do this is to use only a portion of the cytoplasm for the mitochondrial gene correction. To do this, specialists inject only part of the cytoplasm from a healthy donor egg into a recipient egg with mitochondrial gene defects. This procedure is called ooplasmic transfer. Since only a portion of the material from the donor egg is present in the recipient egg, it seems that the ethical problem is solved, and the mother is the woman from whom the recipient egg originates.

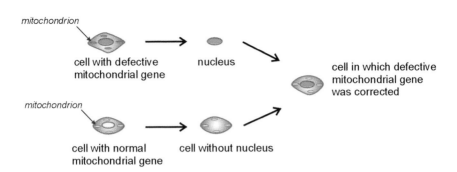

Fig. 1.3   Correction of mitochondrial gene defects. Whole mitochondria carrying a defective gene are replaced, instead of the replacement of just a defective gene alone. Only the nucleus from the egg carrying a defective mitochondrial gene is used, while the rest of the cell is disposed of. Then the nucleus from the egg carrying normal mitochondrial genes is taken out, and replaced with the nucleus taken from the defective cells in which the mitochondrial gene was defective. Now, who is the mother of the new egg?

Future

Gene therapy has already succeeded in the fight against several diseases, and is very close to being widely used in medical practice. Nevertheless, technical problems and safety issues associated with the gene delivery are still great concerns. The improvement of currently existing techniques, however, is definitely possible and will be beneficial. In addition, new techniques, which will continue to facilitate gene therapy, are being developed.

The latest new development is known as short (or small) interfering RNA (siRNA) technology. This technique is based on cell defense mechanisms against viruses, which employ production of siRNA molecules to inactivate viruses. siRNA molecules have the property to initiate the degradation of RNA in the cell that matches their sequence. Consequently, any RNA that matches the injected (foreign) RNAs are degraded and can no longer be used for protein synthesis, turning off the gene (siRNA) that was targeted. This phenomenon can be selectively used to silence the expression of harmful genes. For example, it can be used to silence the gene causing Huntington's disease. Mutations in this gene, called the huntingtin gene, cause production of an abnormal protein that leads to brain damage. Thus, siRNA matching the mutated gene may potentially be used to slow the production of the harmful protein, and to slow

Huntington's disease. SiRNA techniques can also be used to silence viral infections, such as the HIV virus.

All current gene therapy trials involve somatic (non-sex) cells. Germ-line therapy is more technically complex than somatic therapy, and its consequences are more far-reaching. Germ-line therapy would forever change not only the genes of the patient, but also the genes of the descendants of the patient. No germ-line therapy trials have been approved for humans yet, but as the technology becomes safer, germ-line therapy stands to become very useful, at least for the correction of life-threatening defects. On the other hand, germ-line therapy may also have positive implications for future generations. Since defects will be corrected in germ-line cells, they will not be passed on to the next generations and, theoretically, genetic defects will occur less and less in future generations. Will they disappear? Probably not, because new mutations and aberrations always occur in cells as part of natural life.

Gene therapy is based on knowing each gene in the human genome, as well as on our understanding of what it does and how it works. Unfortunately, only a limited percentage of human genes is currently well-analyzed, and most of them have not been identified yet. To accelerate research in this field, human genome programs were launched around the globe, with the largest centers in the US, Europe, and Japan. It is hoped that within the next decade, science will be able to identify all human genes, as well as their main functions. Such knowledge would provide a solid ground for using gene therapy to treat any human genetic disorder. However, considering that genes comprise only 3% of the human genome, will this be sufficient? We do not know yet, but it is doubtful.

References

1. Friedmann T, Roblin R. (1972) Gene therapy for human genetic disease? *Science* **175**: 949–55.
2. Naam R. (2005) *More Than Human: Embracing the Promise of Biological Enhancement.* Broadway Books, New York.

3. Gene Therapy Clinical Trials Worldwide Database. (2012) *The Journal of Gene Medicine.*

4. Hacein-Bey-Abina S., *et al.* (2003) LMO2-associated clonal T cell proliferation in two patients after gene therapy for SCID-X1. *Science* **302:** 415–9.

5. Pearson S, Jia H, Kandachi K. (2004) China approves first gene therapy. *Nat Biotechnol* **22:** 3–4.

6. Foust KD, *et al.* (2009) Intravascular AAV9 preferentially targets neonatal neurons and adult astrocytes. *Nat Biotechnol* **27:** 59–65.

7. Ferrua F, Brigida I, Aiuti A. (2010) Update on gene therapy for adenosine deaminase-deficient severe combined immunodeficiency. *Curr Opin Allergy Clin Immunol* **10:** 551–6.

8. Check E. (2004) Gene therapists hopeful as trials resume with childhood disease. *Nature* **429:** 587.

9. Fischer A, Hacein-Bey-Abina S, Cavazzana-Calvo M. (2010) 20 years of gene therapy for SCID. *Nat Immunol* **11:** 457–60.

10. Rosenberg T. (2011) The Man Who Had HIV and Now Does Not. *New York Magazine,* May 29, 2011.

11. Coghlan A. (2012) Blood tests won't stop gene cheats. *New Scientist,* March 17, 2012.

CHAPTER 2

Genetic Engineering

Definition

Genetic engineering is the gene manipulation technology that aims to create organisms with unnatural properties. This technology allows genes to be mixed from species that cannot normally breed. For example, genetic engineering makes it possible to "transplant" genes from a fish into the genome of a tomato. This is what distinguishes genetic engineering from gene therapy. Gene therapy simply restores altered/mutated genes to their normal state. Also, while gene therapy is exclusively (at least for now) applied to humans, genetic engineering is not performed on humans at all (at least for now). So far, genetic engineering has been widely used to create new crops and foods. It has been also used by the pharmaceutical industry to produce new drugs. Lately, however, concerns have been raised in many countries (especially in Europe) regarding the safety of genetically engineered foods. Thus, the prospects of using this technology in the food industry do not look very bright at this point. Medical applications of this technology, on the other hand, are still in the very early stages and hold great potential. In this chapter, the focus is primarily on the medical aspects of genetic engineering.

History

The first genetic engineering procedures were performed in 1972,[1] when scientists in the US developed recombinant DNA technology, allowing specific genes to be cut and recombined in novel ways (see Fig. 2.1).

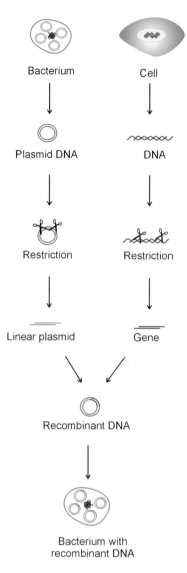

Fig. 2.1   Principles of recombinant DNA technology. This technology allows one to multiply (to clone) a gene of interest. DNA is first isolated from donor cells, and a gene of interest is cut out from DNA using special proteins, which are called restriction enzymes. Then, the gene is inserted into plasmids that are naturally found in bacteria. By cutting DNA, restriction enzymes produce "sticky ends" that allow DNA to stick the gene into plasmids. Plasmids that carry the gene (recombinant plasmids) then can infect bacteria and multiply.

When a gene from another species is inserted into the host, the resulting organism is called transgenic. The first organisms created using genetic engineering were bacteria in 1973, and the first genetically engineered mammals were mice in 1974. When genetic engineering was first developed, the public and the media expressed caution and fear, prompting governments around the world to impose strict rules regarding permissible applications. The excitement then cooled down, and guidelines were relaxed. In 1980, a US Supreme Court ruling allowed for filing patents on genetically engineered living things. In the same year, the first genetically modified organism was patented. It was a bacterium, which had been modified to break down oil.

Soon thereafter, genetically modified organisms, such as bacteria and plants, were approved for release into the environment. In 1978, the biotech company Genentech announced the laboratory production of the first genetically engineered drug, insulin,[2] and a few years later the drug was approved for medical treatments (see more details below).

Many crops, foods, and drugs have been created and sold around the globe using this technology since then. However, progress is slow, and without the spectacular imaginings, such as "super foods" and "Frankenstein weeds" that were at first pictured by sensationalist journalists. As the sensation created by the media hysteria has vanished, instead of voicing concerns, now the public asks if perhaps genetic engineering was oversold. The correct answer is probably "no." Albeit slowly, this technology continues to develop. It does not just happen overnight, and genetic engineering can still deliver on many promises, even making what before seemed impossible come true. Some of the greatest promises of genetic engineering are in the pharmaceutical industry, where many new recombinant biopharmaceutical products are being developed against chronic diseases, such as arthritis and cancer.

Principles

The most useful application of genetic engineering in medicine is in the production of drugs. Principles of this technology are very similar to those

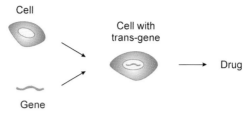

Fig. 2.2   Production of drugs using genetic engineering. A gene that produces a specific drug is isolated and transferred into the cells of interest. Drugs are then synthesized in these cells, isolated, and purified.

of gene therapy (Fig. 2.2). Briefly, a gene of interest has to be isolated and then delivered into the appropriate cells, as described in Chapter 1. New techniques, however, are being developed, and this technology seems to be entering a new, exciting phase. Until recently, genes could only be synthesized using naturally existing gene templates. In addition, only short (no longer than 100 bases) DNA fragments could be synthetically produced. The average size of a gene, however, is more than 1,000 bases. Recently, techniques that allow for the synthesis of DNA molecules stretching for thousands of bases have been developed. This enables the synthesis of full-sized genes and even whole chromosomes; hence, existing or non-existing genes and genomes can be synthesized in laboratories. This opens up a whole new era in genetic engineering, and the first step has already been made. In 2010, scientists at the J. Craig Venter Institute in the US created the world's first synthetic life form: a bacterial cell in which its own genome was discarded and replaced with a chemically synthesized one.[3]

Technical Problems

Genetic engineering and gene therapy are similar technologies and, therefore, they carry similar problems. However, genetic engineering has some specific problems:

(1) **Gene Expression Levels** — Medical-related genetic engineering has some specific applications, such as drug production. In this case, a gene

that encodes a drug must be expressed in the host cells at maximum levels, because the higher the expression level, the higher the amount of the drug produced, and the more of a drug is produced, the cheaper it becomes.

Gene expression is regulated by DNA segments called promoters, which are usually located upstream of the gene's coding sequence. Different promoters initiate gene expression at varying levels. Promoters isolated from viruses are the most frequently used in genetic engineering. They allow the expression of a gene of interest at 1,000 times higher than normal levels. Cells, however, sense foreign bodies and defend themselves against them (especially when numbers of foreign bodies are high). As a result, cells can block the expression of foreign genes and "silence" the trans-genes (foreign genes).

(2) **Allergic Reactions** — Another problem is that some genetically engineered drugs cause allergic immune reactions, which can be potentially fatal. Reasons for this are not yet understood. Possibly, this is due to the fact that such drugs are created by the expression of human genes in bacterial or animal cells. The problem is that after genes are expressed and proteins are assembled from amino acids (as shown in Fig 1.1), the process is not quite yet finished. Proteins very often undergo additional chemical modifications within cells, and these modifications can turn proteins active, inactive, or even harmful. Since human proteins are synthesized in non-human cells, their modifications could end up being incorrect, and thus render them allergic and harmful. Unfortunately, these processes are complex and currently very little understood.

(3) **Drug Resistance** — Additional health problems related to this technology are associated with genetically engineered crops and foods. While trans-genes are transferred into cells, not every cell takes them up and, in most cases, one cannot recognize which cells are actually transgenic and which are not. In order to recognize transgenic cells, scientists attach a marker gene to a trans-gene. The attached marker genes are usually antibiotic resistance genes. They are designed to select transgenic cells through their ability to survive in an environment containing antibiotics against which marker genes were used. As a result, transgenic crops carry not only trans-genes, but also marker antibiotic resistant genes, which creates a

problem. When humans or animals eat transgenic crops, antibiotic resist-ant genes can be absorbed by bacteria that live in the stomach, which can make these bacteria resistant against antibiotics. Thus, genetically engi-neered foods can promote antibiotic resistance in bacteria, which makes it difficult to kill these bacteria and treat diseases that they cause. Considering that antibiotics resistance due to incorrect use or an over-use of antibiotics in medical practice and agriculture is already a threat to public health, using antibiotic resistant genes as markers in genetic engi-neering represents an additional danger. Thus, many specialists endorse a ban on their use in the production of genetically engineered foods.

Applications

Genetic engineering is widely used to produce new crops, foods and drugs. Since this book is focused on medical issues, it mostly describes its applications in the production of drugs. Genetically engineered foods, however, can have adverse effects on health and therefore will also briefly be discussed.

(1) **Crops and Foods** — Genetic engineering was very successfully used to produce plants with desired traits. To do this, genes that are responsible for certain desirable traits were isolated (mostly from bacteria) and trans-ferred into plant cells. Most of the crops (about 85%) were engineered to be resistant against herbicides (chemicals that kill plants) or against pesti-cides (chemicals that kill insects). The remainder of the desired traits include increased resistance to viral diseases or the increased quality of plants, such as longer shelf life, increased vitamin content, and others. Transgenic plants became widely cultivated in the US where, for example, about 55% of all soy and cotton plants are genetically engineered.

In addition to plants, some animals have also been genetically engi-neered. For example, salmon has been modified to produce high levels of growth hormone, which makes the fish grow faster, and thus cheaper to raise.

Introduction of such new species has reduced food costs. Unfortunately, in most cases, trans-genes have negatively affected the quality of food, or even made the food unsafe for human health. For example, genetically engineered soybeans, for some reason, have lower amounts of phytoestrogen compounds, which are believed to protect against heart disease and cancer. Tomatoes, engineered to have a longer storage time without spoiling, have lost taste (and probably some chemicals, such as antioxidants, that benefit human health) when compared to non-genetically engineered tomatoes.

Introduction of foreign genes into plants can cause even more serious consequences. It can induce plant cells to produce allergenic and toxic substances. For example, products made from soybeans carrying the transgene from the Brazil nut plant can cause potentially fatal allergic reactions. Genetically engineered potatoes, as shown in experiments with rats, have adverse effects on the immune system, brain, kidney and other organs, suggesting that these potatoes can be hazardous to human health. Alarmingly, a recent report shows that genetically modified corn can cause tumors and severe damage to the pituitary gland, kidneys, and liver in rats.[4]

(2) **Drugs** — What are drugs? Sometimes, they are simple non-organic chemicals. However, more often, they are complex organic molecules. Simple molecules can usually be synthesized in factories. Most large organic molecules, however, are so complex that they cannot be artificially synthesized, and before genetic engineering was developed, they were usually extracted from human or animal corpses. Drug extraction from corpse tissue, however, poses two major problems: (i) very often, the amount of the molecules of interest is very low and, therefore, a huge amount of corpse material is required in order to extract sufficient quantities of the drug. As a result, the drug becomes expensive; (ii) corpses might contain dangerous substances, such as viruses, which can be hazardous and even fatal if a drug was not sufficiently purified after extraction. Genetic engineering is now solving both of these problems. Instead of synthesizing drugs in factories, biotech companies now engineer animals that can produce drugs in large quantities in their blood, milk, urine, etc., from which the drugs can then be purified. Astonishingly, one single genetically engineered cow or pig can produce as much of a drug of interest as an entire factory! Simpler organisms, or even just cells grown in culture dishes under laboratory conditions can also be used as a "factory" for

producing genetically engineered drugs. For example, insect larvae, fungi, *E. coli* bacteria (found normally in the digestive system), as well as isolated human cells are used for these purposes. As a result, the production costs and the danger of drug contamination have been dramatically reduced. Moreover, many of the new life-saving drugs that were previously impossible to manufacture have become widely available. Examples of some of these drugs include insulin analogs (please see below). Drugs produced in this manner (by genetic engineering techniques) are often called biotech drugs, biologic agents, biopharmaceuticals, or recombinant DNA drugs. Scientists are currently analyzing hundreds of new biotech drugs developed using genetic engineering. Presently, global sales of genetically engineered drugs exceed $30 billion per year, and are growing nearly 10% a year. Below, we will demonstrate two of the most significant examples of how genetic engineering revolutionized the treatment of diseases.

(A) *Insulin* — Insulin was the first genetically engineered medicine. Bringing this drug to medical practices paved the way for regulation, commerce, and adjusting social issues for the rest of the genetically engineered drugs to come. Why insulin? Quite simply, because there is a huge demand for this medicine. Insulin is a hormone produced by the pancreas that regulates blood glucose levels. When its levels become abnormally low, people develop a common type of diabetes (type I diabetes). Of note, when a person's cells fail to respond to insulin, the person can develop another common type of diabetes (type II). Patients with low insulin levels, or those who fail to respond to normal levels of insulin, can be treated with daily injections of this hormone and live normally. Before genetic engineering, insulin was produced by extraction and purification of this hormone from slaughtered animals, mainly from cattle and pigs. In 1978, the human gene encoding insulin was isolated and cloned in *E. coli* bacteria (as shown in Fig. 2.1). It was done jointly by the then-fledging company Genentech and The City of Hope National Medical Center in the US. Soon after, the pharmaceutical company Lilly, a leader in insulin manufacturing at that time, licensed this recombinant insulin and brought it to the market. Genetically engineered insulin was first approved for treatment in 1982 in the UK and soon after in other countries. More recently, insulin analogs that differ in a few amino acids from original insulin were created to control its activity and stability. For example, some insulin analogs last for up to 24 hours in the body, so only one injection is need daily. Today, insulin products generate huge revenues — for example, more than $3 billion is generated annually in sales for the company Novo alone.

(B) *Blood factor VIII* — Factor VIII is a protein that is essential for blood clotting. Lack of or low levels of this protein in the blood causes hemophilia A, which is the most common form of bleeding disorder. Traditionally, this disorder was treated using factor VIII isolated from the plasma of donor blood. In the 1980s, however, it was discovered that plasma can transmit fatal viral infections, such as HIV. Since then, plasma undergoes special treatments to eliminate this infection. Nevertheless, the danger still remains, and currently, there is a great deal of concern about transmission of other viral infections, such as Creutzfeldt–Jakob disease. This prompted scientists to search for artificial sources of factor VIII. This protein, however, is large and too complex to make in a tube. The solution came when the gene that encodes for the factor VIII was identified. In 1989, the gene was cloned and placed into mammalian cells, where it could be expressed at high levels.[5] Soon after, this recombinant protein was successfully used for the treatment of people with hemophilia. Since then, factor VIII has become a good example of how the most complex proteins can be manufactured through recombinant DNA technology.

Controversies

As discussed in Chapter 1, genetic engineering does not directly deal with the human genome. The technology that does so is called gene therapy. Since genetic engineering does not involve genetic manipulations of humans by definition, it does not raise big controversies.

Future

One of the most promising applications of genetic engineering in medicine is in the production of antibodies. Currently, antibodies represent over 30% of biopharmaceuticals tested in clinical trials. Antibodies can be especially valuable in the treatment of cancers, arthritis and other chronic diseases.

What are antibodies? They are proteins produced by cells that serve to recognize and eliminate any foreign substances in the body. These foreign substances can be bacteria, viruses, abnormal cells (such as cancer cells), and in some cases, large biological molecules (sometimes even drugs). Scientists call these foreign substances "antigens." Antigens can be harmful, and one's survival depends on antibodies. Normally, all cells have special marks that tell the immune system: "I belong to your own body, don't touch me." Immune cells constantly check the body for these marks and, if they find something that is not correctly marked, they produce antibodies that attach themselves to the foreign substance. This attachment either inactivates the substance or marks it for elimination by immune cells. It is very important that the antibody does the following: (1) recognize a foreign object and (2) does not recognize and attach to the body's own cells (as this would cause destruction of the body). This can be a challenge for the immune system, and when our own immune system fails to act appropriately, modern medicine can help by producing and injecting the appropriate antibody.

There are two types of antibodies — monoclonal and polyclonal. Polyclonal antibodies are derived from different cell lines, while monoclonal antibodies are derived from the generation of one single cell (one clone). Since monoclonal antibodies originate from one cell line, they are identical, making them more specific to the antigen. This characteristic renders them the tool of choice in modern medical practice.

Antibodies are an especially promising tool in fighting cancers. Cancerous cells constantly appear in the body, but in most cases, they are recognized and eliminated by the immune system. When any cell becomes cancerous, it either loses proper self markers that normally tell the immune cells that the cell is a part of the body, or it acquires new markers identifying it as a foreign cell. Thus, cells that become cancerous are normally eliminated, keeping cancer away. The problem arises when the immune system becomes weak, or when cell transformation is so masked or unusual that immune cells cannot synthesize the proper antigens. This can be helped by the injection of synthetic antibodies. The trick is to find some special feature of cancer cells, against which the antibody could react. One distinct feature of cancer cells is that they divide indefinitely, and they do not age. Although many normal cells in the body constantly divide, their division number is limited and they are senescent (meaning that they age). Therefore, it is possible that cancerous cells carry specific features, and it is possible that these features can eventually be detected using antibodies. Several antibodies that help in cancer treatment have already been developed. Among others is the anti-CD20 antibody that has revolutionized the treatment of lymphomas, the trastuzumab antibody against breast cancer, and the cetuximab antibody used against colon cancer.

Methods by which antibodies are produced are also evolving and improving. They are normally produced in animals, such as mice and rabbits. Recently, monoclonal antibodies for use against breast and colorectal cancers were successfully produced using genetically engineered tobacco, which simplifies production and makes them cheaper. The success of antibodies in disease treatment depends upon good design. Fortunately, our knowledge about antibody engineering is expanding rapidly. More and more antibodies are becoming useful in treatments, and they may soon revolutionize clinical practice.

References

1. Jackson DA, Symons RH, Berg P. (1972) Biochemical method for inserting new genetic information into DNA of Simian Virus 40: circular SV40 DNA molecules containing lambda phage genes and the galactose operon of *Escherichia coli*. *Proc Natl Acad Sci USA* **69:** 2904–9.
2. Genentech. (1978) First Successful Laboratory Production of Human Insulin Announced. News Release, Sept 6, 1978.
3. Gibson DG, *et al.* (2010) Creation of a bacterial cell controlled by a chemically synthesized genome. *Science* **329:** 52–6.
4. Seralini GE, *et al.* (2012) Long term toxicity of a Roundup herbicide and a Roundup-tolerant genetically modified maize. *Food Chem Toxicol* **50(11):** 4221–31.
5. Kaufman RJ. (1989) Genetic engineering of factor VIII. *Nature* **342:** 207–8.

CHAPTER 3

Human Cloning

Definition

Cloning is the creation of an identical copy of something. The term clone is derived from the Greek language. It means "twig," which refers to the process by which a new plant can be created from a twig. Creating plants from twigs, or cloning of plants, has been known since ancient times. Many plants can be grown simply from one single leaf, a piece of stem, or a piece of root. For example, potato cultivation is nothing other than cloning using roots. Grapes can also be cloned, and some European grape cultivars represent clones that have now been propagated for millennia. Human cloning, however, is not that easy. A piece of human finger or ear left on the soil cannot just grow into a human. For many years now, scientists have tried to understand how to clone humans, and it seems like success is not too far away. One by one, several mammalian species have now been cloned: sheep, cat, horse, and even a monkey.

Depending on the purpose, human cloning can be defined as either reproductive or therapeutic. Reproductive cloning is the process of creating a genetically identical copy of an existing human. Therapeutic cloning is the process of creating body parts or organs that genetically match that of an existing person. Until recently, cloning was only intended to be reproductive. Now, with new developments in stem cell technology, therapeutic cloning aimed to repair human tissues and organs is being developed. In therapeutic cloning, a cloned human embryo is not grown into a full human, but rather, is used to isolate stem cells. Stem cells are then used to grow tissues or organs that genetically match the person from which they originate. Therapeutic cloning is a very promising tool in modern medicine, as it can solve two major medical problems: (1) immune rejection of transplanted organs (since transplanted organs or body parts are genetically identical with the patient, they will not be rejected by the immune system of the person to which they are transplanted); (2) it can eliminate the shortage of organs available for transplantation.

History

Humans are among the most complex organisms and, thusly, they are among the most difficult to clone. In addition, human cloning raises moral, ethical, religious, and all other kinds of problems. The foundation of the science used in human cloning was derived by cloning simple organisms. The first animal ever cloned was a tadpole, in 1952. However, human cloning was not feasible until the first mammal was cloned. It was the sheep, in 1996, named Dolly, which was created by scientists from the UK.[1] Dolly was a hallmark in the history of cloning, because it demonstrated that genomes from specialized somatic cells of mammals can be reprogrammed to generate an entire organism. Several other mammals, including mice, cats, and the rhesus monkey, have been cloned. Thousands of cloned animals have already been produced around the world, and many scientists now believe that human cloning will be possible very soon. Moreover, claims of human cloning have even been made. For example, a company known as Clonaid, which is associated with a religion called Raelism, claimed in 2002 that it successfully cloned a human being. By 2004, this company claimed that 13 children had been already cloned. However, no evidence of this was ever shown. More claims have been made by others, but similar to the Clonaid case, no evidence of this has been produced.

Nevertheless, the first step in human cloning has already been made. In 2001, a privately funded company called Advanced Cell Technology, based in the US, announced the first cloned human embryo.[2] Later, human embryo cloning was performed by several other teams of scientists; however, these embryos did not survive for a long time (see below).

Principles

Each and every cell in the body (except certain cells in the immune system) contains the same genetic material, and theoretically, almost any cell in the body can be used for cloning. However, two types of cells can be found in the body — germ and somatic cells. The only germ cells in the human body are either egg cells found in women, or sperm cells found in men. The rest of the cells in our bodies are somatic. The difference between germ cells and somatic cells is that germ cells have only one set of genes (see Chapter 1 for more information about genes), while somatic cells have two sets (a duplicated gene set). When the egg merges with the sperm cell, two sets of genes are formed (which are duplicates of each other) creating a somatic cell, and the merged cell then divides to produce more somatic cells. However, if the nucleus of the egg (which contains one set of genes) is replaced with the nucleus of any somatic cell (which contains a duplicated set of genes), the resulting egg cell can divide and grow into a full human being without ever being fertilized by a sperm cell. This technique is employed in human cloning, and could be done through the procedure known as nuclear transplantation, or somatic cell nuclear transfer (Fig. 3.1).

Although genetic material in all somatic cells is the same, differentiated somatic cells look different, and they perform different functions. This is because only a fraction of the genes, at any given moment, is active in cells. Genes regulate each other, and they can also be turned "on" or "off" by environmental signals. When the nucleus from a somatic cell is transplanted into an egg cell, its genes are reprogrammed by the environment of the egg to form a new human being. These signals are incorporated in egg cells. What are those signals? Science does not yet have an answer. If they were known, there would be no need for the transplantation of somatic nuclear DNA into an egg for cloning. Instead, one could just use these signals for cloning human beings from any somatic cell.

The procedure for reproductive and therapeutic cloning begins similarly — the nucleus of an egg is replaced with the nucleus from a somatic cell (Fig. 3.1). The reconstructed egg is then treated with either an electric current, or with chemicals, to initiate cell division and the formation of

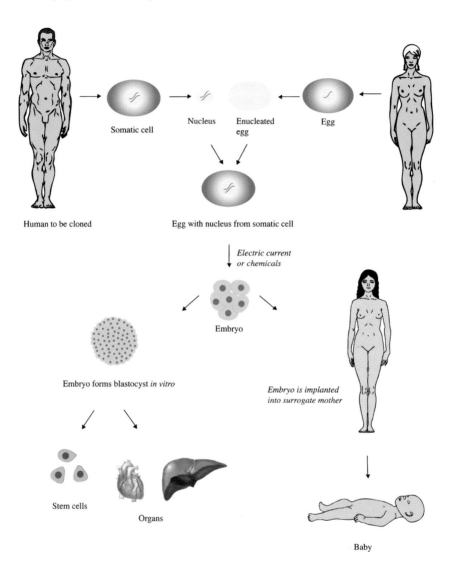

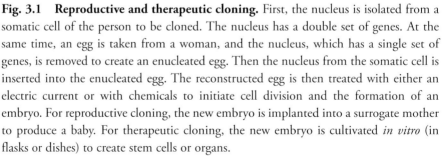

Fig. 3.1   Reproductive and therapeutic cloning. First, the nucleus is isolated from a somatic cell of the person to be cloned. The nucleus has a double set of genes. At the same time, an egg is taken from a woman, and the nucleus, which has a single set of genes, is removed to create an enucleated egg. Then the nucleus from the somatic cell is inserted into the enucleated egg. The reconstructed egg is then treated with either an electric current or with chemicals to initiate cell division and the formation of an embryo. For reproductive cloning, the new embryo is implanted into a surrogate mother to produce a baby. For therapeutic cloning, the new embryo is cultivated *in vitro* (in flasks or dishes) to create stem cells or organs.

an embryo. For reproductive cloning, the new embryo is then implanted into a surrogate mother to produce a baby. For therapeutic cloning, the new embryo is cultivated *in vitro* (in flasks or dishes) to create stem cells and then organs.

Technical Problems

The procedure of human cloning is challenging. For example, when Advanced Cell Technology claimed the first cloned 100% human embryo, eight nuclear transplantations had to be performed. Only three out of eight eggs began dividing, and only one egg was able to divide into a six-celled embryo before stopping. It must be noted here that no baby was produced, and there is still a very long way between a six-celled embryo and a baby. Eggs can lose their ability to divide due to the removal of nuclei,[3] which probably damages other cellular components. From experiments with animal cloning, it is estimated that an average of more than 100 nuclear transfer procedures are necessary to produce one viable embryo. To produce Dolly, 277 eggs were used to produce 29 embryos, of which only one produced the adult animal!

Not only is the procedure of human cloning challenging, but the very idea of human cloning is questionable for the following reasons:

(1) Only the nucleus is used to clone a human being, while the rest of the cell originates from another person (please see Fig. 3.1). As shown in Chapter 1, not all genes are contained in nuclei. A small portion (about 0.1%) of human genetic material is stored in the mitochondria, which are located in the cytoplasm of cells. This means that the mitochondrial genes of a cloned human being would originate from another person, and the clone would only be 99.99% identical to the original. Keeping this in mind, it appears that women will have cloning advantages compared to men. This is because men do not have egg cells, and the egg for cloning a male should originate from a female, which is a different human being. In the case of female cloning, it is possible to use the egg cell and the nucleus from the same person, which makes the mitochondrial genome of the clone and the original identical.

(2) Cells that build the human body constantly mutate and, therefore, theoretically, there may be no cells with 100% identical nuclear genomes in our bodies. This means that even the nuclear genome of a clone will always be slightly different when compared to the genome of the original.

(3) Cells in cloned embryos are unstable. This is because during cloning, nuclear genes are transferred from one cell into another cell, and therefore, into a completely different environment. As the result, many genes in the reconstructed cells become deregulated and function abnormally, which often leads either to the rejection of cloned embryos by the surrogate mother, or to the transformation of cells into tumors.

(4) For as yet unknown reasons, cloned animals usually have high rates of deformities and disabilities. They also age faster than the original species. This might be due to the fact that cells from adult organisms are used for cloning, and it is possible that such cells "remember" their age and are pre-programmed for faster aging.

Despite of all these difficulties, it is widely believed that cloning procedures will be adjusted, and human beings can be cloned soon.

Applications

One of the most plausible applications of reproductive cloning would be the creation of babies for infertile families. This would be a significant contribution to society, because about 1 out of 12 families is currently affected by infertility. At this time, however, reproductive cloning seems like a distant future. In contrast, therapeutic cloning may be practiced soon, and it can be applied as follows:

(1) **Organ Transplantation** — Organs required for transplantation can be produced using cloning. Cloning could provide a never-ending supply of donor organs. Moreover, cloned organs will be genetically matched to the recipient, and the danger of rejection of transplanted organs will be eliminated. No longer will patients have to wait until

a donor dies to obtain a transplant; no longer will someone have to donate one kidney (humans have two kidneys) to save his or her relative or friend. Many lives, otherwise lost due to the shortage of available organs, will be saved. Moreover, brand new organs will be available. They could be better quality than organs now available for transplantation, which sometimes have a short lifetime. However, there is no data on the quality of cloned organs as yet.

Cloning such organs as the heart, liver, and kidneys should become possible. Cloning can also revolutionize cosmetic procedures. For example, it should be possible to clone human hair and thus to treat baldness. Since hair is one of the simplest organs, it will probably be one of the first human organs cloned. The first step of cloning organs is already done — cloning human embryos, from which any organ can later be produced by this embryo. However, it might take many years before growing functional organs from embryos becomes a reality.

(2) **Regeneration of Damaged Tissues** — In some cases, when organs are only locally damaged, it would be possible to restore their functions using stem cells, which can be produced using therapeutic cloning (see Fig. 3.1). In other cases, such as nerve damage, transplantation is not possible. However, repair using stem cells looks feasible in these cases. Scientists have already learned how to produce stem cells using cloning. Now, they are working to figure out how to repair nerve, brain, skin, and other tissues using such cells.

(3) **Xenotransplantation** — Animals and plants could also be cloned for medical purposes. For example, human organs can be replaced by organs from cloned animals (xenotransplantation). To avoid possible rejection, animals can be genetically modified to "knock-out" genes that are responsible for triggering the immune rejection. Then, such animals can be cloned and farmed for transplant organs. The most suitable candidates for such work are pigs. Why pigs? Because of all the animal species that have been successfully cloned so far, organs from pigs are the most similar to human ones. They have already been used (for example, heart) for transplantation into humans. Organs from primates would be genetically closer to human organs;

however, primates are much more difficult to clone. Moreover, using primates for such purposes would probably cause controversies and protests. How close are transplanted organs from cloned pigs to reality? It seems close. In 2002, scientists reported the production of the first "knock-out" pigs, which lack a gene involved in transplant rejection.[4] Unfortunately, there are about 600 genes responsible for tissue matching. Although it may not be necessary to knock them all out to prevent transplant rejection, it would probably be necessary to knock out at least several of them.

Controversies

Both reproductive and therapeutic human cloning raise sharp criticisms. The very idea of human cloning is controversial, and the answer to the question of whether it should be permitted depends on religion and beliefs. For example, the Roman Catholic Church is clearly opposed to any kind of human cloning. The Jewish religion takes the position that human cloning can be justified in some circumstances. Islamic religious thinkers have not come yet to an agreement about whether human cloning should be permitted. Of course, the acceptability of human cloning also depends on motivations and intentions. Human cloning can be used for wrong or evil purposes in many ways. Nevertheless, even if one agrees with the very idea that human cloning should be permitted for the right causes, many concerns and problems still remain unresolved:

(1) **Reliability and Safety of the Procedure** — As mentioned above, it is estimated that an average of more than 100 nuclear transfer procedures (and eggs) are necessary to produce one viable animal embryo. Since human cloning is more complex, it might require many more procedures, and even more eggs would be wasted. Therefore, many people believe that, at the current state of the technology, human cloning would be wasteful and unethical.

(2) **Safety of the Procedure** — When animals are successfully cloned, for reasons that are not yet clear, they have high rates of deformities and disabilities. In addition, they appear to be non-viable over a normal life-span. They age faster and they die prematurely. There is no

reason to believe that human cloning will not encounter similar problems. Considering the complexity of the human brain, cloning would, most likely, encounter even more problems. With so many unknowns, human cloning is very risky and, therefore, unethical at this time.

(3) **Genetic Diversity** — During the normal process of conception of a baby, the genome of a male is mixed with the genome of a female. In cloned babies, almost the entire set of genetic material would originate from only one person, which would reduce the genetic diversity of such humans. Genetic diversity helps us to adapt to living conditions and it drives our evolution. Therefore, large-scale cloning might make humans more fragile and less adaptable to the environment.

(4) **Parental Issues** — For cloning, the nucleus of the egg is taken out and replaced with the nucleus from a somatic cell. The individual from whom the nucleus originates is considered the parent. However, the individual from whom the egg is taken might also have parental rights. In addition, the clone technically represents a delayed twin of the individual from whom the nucleus was taken, rather than his/her child. Will this affect the relationship between the parent and the cloned child? This has never happened before, and we do not know what emotional problems this can raise.

(5) **Sex Issues** — Only egg, but no sperm cells, are required for cloning. If cloning is performed on a large scale, men will not be necessary for reproduction and could be allowed to die off, and only women would be left.

(6) **Soul** — Some believe that souls exist, and that the soul is formed when a sperm cell fertilizes an egg. Since cloning does not involve sperm cells, there is a concern that cloned humans might have no soul.

Although reproductive human cloning is still in the distant future, therapeutic cloning might be just a few years away. For therapeutic cloning, embryos are created and then destroyed and used as repair material. This raises a very sharp question — is destroying the embryos equal to killing human beings? Some people think that an egg with a somatic nucleus is already a human being, while others do not. Accordingly, some governments currently allow therapeutic cloning while others do not. For example, the US bans both reproductive and therapeutic cloning, while the UK prohibits reproductive cloning but allows therapeutic cloning. The United Nations has discussed this issue, but did not adopt a clear resolution. The resolution speaks against reproductive cloning, but it is non-binding and it does not oblige states to enforce it. However, progress in science, especially in stem cell research, may soften or even eliminate some controversies. For example, it may not be necessary to destroy embryos for therapeutic cloning in the future. It has been found that it is possible to create embryonic stem cells from a single cell (called blasto-mere) of an embryo, and such an operation does not interfere with the embryo's further development.[5]

Future

Whether reproductive cloning is possible still remains to be seen. It is clear, however, that given the present state of the technology, there is no way to clone humans reliably and safely. In the future, as the reliability and safety issues improve, it is logical to expect that opposition to human cloning might ease. However, it will take a long time before reproductive human cloning becomes a reality.

In contrast, therapeutic human cloning is very close to being practi-cally applied. Human embryos have already been cloned, and it is prob-ably a matter of a few years before organs and tissues from cloned human embryos are produced. Currently, the demand for transplant organs far outstrips the supply. Some patients have to wait for many years before organs become available, and some patients die before that. Therefore, the demand for cloned organs and tissues will be large. This raises the question — if organs are cloned, where will all eggs for the cloning come from? Probably, not every woman will donate her egg cells for the pur-pose of therapeutic cloning. Some women, however, may donate many eggs and collections of them might be created. Most likely, therapeutic cloning will be done at special facilities, and organ/tissue farming will be created.

References

1. Campbell KH, McWhir J, Ritchie WA, Wilmut I. (1996) Sheep cloned by nuclear transfer from a cultured cell line. *Nature* **380:** 64–6.
2. Cibelli JB, Lanza RP, West MD, Ezzell C. (2001) The First Human Cloned Embryo. *Scientific American,* Nov 24, 2001.
3. Noggle S, *et al.* (2011) Human oocytes reprogram somatic cells to a pluripotent state. *Nature* **478:** 70–5.
4. Lai L, *et al.* (2002) Production of alpha-1,3-galactosyltransferase knockout pigs by nuclear transfer cloning. *Science* **295:** 1089–92.
5. Klimanskaya I, Chung Y, Becker S, *et al.* (2006) Human embryonic stem cell lines derived from single blastomeres. *Nature* **444:** 481–5.

CHAPTER 4

Stem Cell Technology

Definition

Cells in the body carry out specific functions. For example, red blood cells bind molecules of oxygen and transport them to other cells, muscle cells contract and expand to facilitate movement, and so on. Some cells, such as neuronal cells, do not divide, while others, such as skin cells, can divide to renew worn out or damaged tissue. Dividing cells in the body, however, have a finite ability to multiply and are called senescent cells. For example, they can be programmed to divide 30 or 40 times, after which they age and die. In contrast, stem cells, a different class of cells which are also found in special areas of the body, can multiply an unlimited number of times. Similarly, cancer cells can also multiply an unlimited number of times, and their uncontrolled division causes trouble. The division of stem cells, however, is controlled, and when divided, they undergo transformation from unspecialized cells into cells with specialized functions (Fig. 4.1). Thus, we can define stem cells as cells that can renew themselves and give rise to specialized cells.

Stem cells have different potencies and they can be: (a) totipotent, which means that they can form any cell type including an embryonic one; (b) pluripotent, which means that they can form any cell type, except for an embryonic one; (c) multipotent/oligopotent, which means that they can produce only several closely related families of cells; and (d) unipotent, which means that they can form only one type, their own cell type.

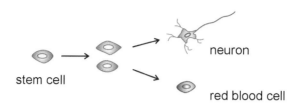

Fig. 4.1   Stem cells. Stem cells can multiply and give rise to cells with specialized functions, such as neurons and red blood cells.

History

Stem cells have been known in science for several decades. They can be found not only in humans, but also in animals and plants. Although stem cell technology began to develop just a decade ago or so, their existence was postulated more than a century ago, in 1908, by the Russian histologist A. Maximov. Stem cells have been used to manipulate and regenerate plants for over two decades. In medicine, attention to them began to increase since 1998, when stem cells were isolated from embryos and cultured under laboratory conditions.[1] It soon became clear that stem cells had tremendous potential in medicine, and research in the field began to accelerate. Unfortunately, stem cell applications in medicine raised serious ethical issues, which led to policies permitting only the limited use of embryonic stem cells in most industrialized countries. This has slowed progress, but did not stop it. Progress continues, and new methods that diminish controversies associated with embryonic stem cells have recently been invented.

Principles

Stem cells can be isolated either from adult human bodies or from embryos. Hence, they are called either adult stem cells or embryonic stem cells (ES cells).

(1) **Adult Stem Cells** — Stem cells can be found in our bodies. Most cells in the body wear out on a regular basis and have to be replaced. For example, dandruff on the scalp or peeling skin after a sunburn are nothing other than dead skin cells. Cells in other organs are also constantly renewed,

although we do not see this. Among these are blood cells, muscle cells, and even neuronal cells. These new cells originate from stem cells hidden in adult organs. So far, adult stem cells have been found in several organs — bone marrow, brain, muscle, skin, liver, and others.

Stems cells have the following fundamental properties: (1) they can divide and multiply many times; (2) they have no specific function, except for constant renewal; (3) under certain conditions they can be transformed into specialized cells (this process is called differentiation). For example, stem cells located in the red marrow of bones can give rise to erythrocytes — red blood cells that are able to bind and carry oxygen through the bloodstream (Fig. 4.2). Stem cells located in the olfactory bulb of the brain can give rise to neurons — cells that are able to fire electrochemical signals to other cells. The body uses certain types of adult stem cells to repair particular organs. For example, blood stem cells from bone marrow serve to replace old cells in the blood, while neural stem cells from the olfactory bulb serve to repair the brain. This gives rise to opportunities for their use in medicine. Neural stem cells might be used to repair damaged brain

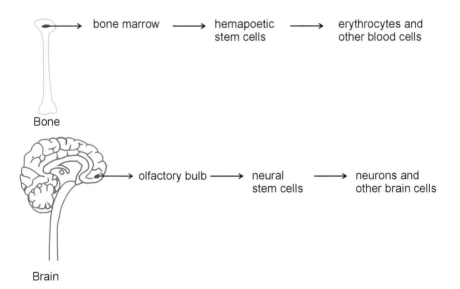

Fig. 4.2   Adult stem cells. Adult stem cells can be found in several organs; for example, in bone marrow and in the brain.

tissue, skin stem cells might be used to repair damaged skin, etc. Blood cells do not originate from neural stem cells, while brain cells do not develop from blood stem cells. Later, we will see that this can be possible under manipulative laboratory conditions.

(2) **Embryonic Stem (ES) Cells** — ES cells are developed from embryos. Each cell of a human embryo is a potential stem cell that can multiply and give rise to a number of different cell types.

Today, when people talk about stem cells, they usually mean ES cells. Most of us do not even suspect that there are other types of stem cells. ES cells raise a lot of controversy, mostly due to ethical questions such as: Is someone killed to develop these cells? Do we have rights to use them at all? But before delving into this problem, we should try to understand what ES cells are. Let us first figure out what an embryo is and what is this thing from which ES cells originate?

An embryo is basically a ball composed of several cells (Fig. 4.3). Where do they come from? They are developed after the merging of a female egg cell with a male sperm cell. The sperm cell penetrates the egg,

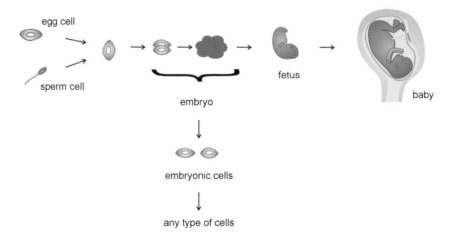

Fig. 4.3   Embryonic stem (ES) cells. ES cells originate from embryos. An embryo is a ball of cells that develops after the merging of a female egg cell with a male sperm cell. Eight weeks after the merging, embryonic cells form a fetus and then a baby.

then the egg and the sperm cell merge and form a single cell, called a zygote. The resulting cell then divides and produces two cells, which by day three divide twice and generate eight cells. Each of the cells at this stage is totipotent — meaning that it can transform into any cell type of the body and produce a full human. The cells continue to divide, and for another seven weeks they are still called an embryo. By the eighth week, they form a structure about 5 cm long, which is no longer called an embryo, but a fetus. The ES cells currently being used in gene therapy are developed from four-to-six day old embryos, which look like hollow balls, called blastocysts. These embryos consist of 50 to 150 cells. They have a diameter of only one-seventh of a millimeter and are almost invisible to the naked eye. ES cells are developed from embryos that were created *in vitro* (meaning artificially in laboratories). The purpose of creating such artificial embryos is to help infertile parents to conceive children. But because many of the artificially created embryos do not survive, and not all of them are able to develop into a baby, laboratories create many embryos, even though a couple is trying to have just one baby. Usually, only one or a few embryos are selected for the family. The rest of them are no longer needed and kept frozen. These embryos that are not needed and would otherwise have been disposed of are used to develop ES cells.

(3) **Adult Stem Cells versus ES Cells** — Until recently, it was believed that adult stem cells were only able to generate certain types of cells to repair designated organs. For example, only neural stem cells (localized in the brain) can produce brain cells and only blood stem cells (localized in bone marrow) can develop into blood cells. It now appears that this might not be true. It was recently discovered that blood stem cells, under certain conditions, can give rise to brain cells as well as to skeletal muscle cells, cardiac muscle cells, and liver cells. Brain stem cells, on the other hand, were recently transformed into blood cells. It seems that all of this depends on the environment in which the stem cells are placed and the signals that they receive. Science must now find the appropriate chemical and physical conditions. This opens up the possibility of tricking adult stem cells into behaving as early embryo cells, which can be transformed to any type of cell. While the majority of the attention is currently focused on ES

cells, such a trick would move adult stem cells onto the front lines of progress, and would probably alleviate the need to use ES cells. Why? Using ES cells has two big problems. First, there are ethical problems, which have forced governments of many industrial countries to limit their use. Adult stem cells, on the other hand, don't raise these kinds of ethical concerns — they originate from the cells of the patient who needs them, and no potential life is terminated. A second problem is biological — ES cells originate from cells other than the patient's and thus, are not genetically identical to the cells of the patient who might need them. As a result, these cells (and tissues or organs created by using them) might be rejected by the patient's body. Adult stem cells, on the other hand, can be taken from the patient's own body, manipulated to produce appropriate cells, tissues or organs, and then transplanted. Since all cells in the body of an individual are genetically identical, they will not be rejected.

The use of adult instead of embryonic stem cells is getting very close to reality. Adult stem cells can be transformed into pluripotent cells by genetic reprogramming, during which specific genes involved in cell division/differentiation are forcefully induced. Such transformed stem cells are called induced pluripotent stem (iPS) cells (see more details below). Scientists are also trying to combine adult and embryonic stem cell approaches. The idea is to take cells from any organ of a patient (they are called somatic cells), and to create from them an embryo using cloning techniques. This embryo could then be used to obtain the genetically identical cells that the patient needs. This approach is called therapeutic cloning. Unfortunately, instead of solving issues, this might create additional problems. The first is, once again, a moral one — does one create life to destroy it? The second is a technical one — it seems that current methods of cloning do not really allow development of a 100% genetically identical human embryo (please see Chapter 3).

Technical Problems

Stem cell technology can make tremendous contributions to the field of regenerative medicine. The general idea of stem cell use in regenerative medicine is simple: Just isolate and transplant them into the tissue that needs to be repaired. This is happening in laboratories so far, and experiments designed to regenerate tissues have been performed at a faster pace than experiments addressing basic stem cell science. However, it soon became clear that many fundamental issues should be addressed before stem cells are used in medical practice. Among them are two main problems: the immune rejection of the transplanted stem cells, and the formation of tumors by the transplanted stem cells.

(1) **Immune Rejection** — The immune system recognizes foreign cells and attacks them, causing the rejection of transplanted cells or organs. Since stem cells usually originate from a source other than one's own body, they will be rejected. Nevertheless, some types of cells are more prone to rejection than others. For example, the risk of rejection of vascular endothelial cells is higher than that for liver cells. Therefore, one approach to avoid rejection could be the isolation and selection of those types of stem cells that induce milder rejection. Such cells can be developed from adult stem cells found in those organs that cause mild immune rejection, such as the liver. Another approach could be modifying stem cells to match them to the patient's immune system, using genetic engineering. Using this technique, it is theoretically possible to introduce or to eliminate genes that encode the proteins that are responsible for immune system recognition. This, however, requires more knowledge than we presently have about genes involved in immune system recognition. Finally, another very promising approach is based on generating stem cells that genetically match the patient's own cells, using the technique called "somatic cell nuclear transfer." In this technique, the stem cell nucleus, which contains the genetic information, is replaced by the nucleus of a somatic cell from the patient. The newly generated stem cell will have genes identical to the patient's genetic material and, theoretically, should not be rejected. However, as mentioned in Chapter 3, cells lose their ability to divide due to replacement of nuclei, and this procedure has a very low success rate.

It appears now that such procedures may no longer be necessary, and it is possible to transform adult human cells into pluripotent stem cells, similar to embryonic stem cells, using genetic reprogramming. At first, such induced pluripotent stem (iPS) cells were produced using mouse cells.[2]

Then, in 2007, one group in Japan[3] and another one in the US[4] independently carried out experiments using somatic cells from human skin. These experiments laid the groundwork for successful experimentations to transform one cell type into virtually any other one. For example, skin cells were recently used to produce functional neurons with this approach.[5] This implies that with proper adjustments, all cells may be able to form all kinds of tissues. Such procedures may eliminate the need of ES cells in regenerative medicine, which would also eliminate moral controversies associated with the use of embryonic stem cells. However, these procedures may also modify the genetic makeup of the transformed cells, causing side effects; thus, they need more adjustments before use in medical practices.

Promising findings were also published by a group of German scientists. This group has demonstrated that cells from an adult human testis can be used to generate embryonic-like stem cells.[6] Such cells would completely match the cells of a person from which they were developed, and this could solve the problem of rejection. In addition, it would make using embryos unnecessary, and it would eliminate controversies associated with their use (see below). However, since the cells are developed from the testis, this will only help men.

(2) **Tumor Formation** — Similar to cancerous cells, stem cells have the potential to divide indefinitely. Stem cells, however, also have the ability to differentiate and to stop dividing. Continued division without differentiation will lead to the formation of tumors. Indeed, experiments with animals have demonstrated that the transplantation of stem cells causes the formation of benign tumors. Injected embryonic stem cells can develop into many different cell types and form tumors called teratoma. This raises the question: Is stem cell transplantation for regenerative purposes possible without the danger of tumor formation? Several possible solutions are currently being explored. One way to solve the problem involves finding appropriate hormones and chemicals to induce transplanted stem cells to differentiate, rather than to form tumors. Another way would be co-transplantation of "inducer tissues" that interact with transplanted stem cells and promote their differentiation. These possibilities are still under experimentation, and more basic knowledge on how the body controls the differentiation of stem cells is needed for future progress.

(3) **Other Problems** — In many cases, stem cell transplantation might be required to restore functions of damaged organs. For example, it might be required to restore the heart tissue that was damaged during a heart attack, or skin damaged by fire. Such damaged tissues are often inflamed and become hostile to transplanted stem cells. The inflammation that creates a hostile environment for transplanted cells can be a serious problem. It is estimated, for example, that up to 95% of the cells currently used for heart failure treatment die before they incorporate into the heart tissue. Another common problem of stem cell therapy is possible bacterial or viral infections that occur during the procedure.

Applications

Tissues and organs routinely use adult stem cells to maintain and repair themselves. In case of accidents or diseases, however, the damage can be too great to be naturally repaired — for example, extensive skin burns caused by fire or nerve damage caused by accidents, which leave people permanently disfigured or paralyzed. Nevertheless, stem cells can be artificially grown in large numbers in the laboratory, differentiated into the appropriate cells, and used to repair damaged organs. Neural stem cells could be used to repair damaged brain tissue, skin stem cells could be used to repair damaged skin, etc. Applications of ES cells look even more promising. These cells are able to develop into virtually any cell in a human body and therefore, theoretically, they can be used to repair any organ. Below are examples of how some diseases could be treated using stem cells:

(1) **Spinal Cord Injury** — This problem is probably one of the first things that comes to mind when thinking of possible stem cell applications. Even a tiny amount of damage to the spinal cord can cause dramatic consequences. A little cut, and a person is paralyzed for a lifetime! So, how could such an injury be fixed? The spinal cord is a bundle of axons, which are nothing more than extensions of neuronal cells that allow them to communicate with each other. A spinal cord injury is just a cut in these extensions that blocks the ability of the neurons to send signals. It is not even a loss of cells. Today, there is great pressure on doctors to apply stem cell techniques to repair such damage. As early as the

year 2000, experiments on animals demonstrated that it is possible. In experiments involving rats, transplanted ES cells could differentiate into neuronal cells, extend their axons and restore the function of a damaged spinal cord. And yet, extrapolating this technology to humans requires a lot of caution, and the efficacy of this therapy is still uncertain. How soon will this technology be used to repair a spinal cord? It seems that it might happen as soon as the next few years, but the serious problems discussed above would still have to be solved. Indeed, the first human trial using stem cells, initiated in the US in 2010 by a privately held company, Geron, had to be discontinued.[7] In this trial, four patients with spinal cord injuries were treated but, for whatever reasons, there were "no signs" that the treatment was helping the patients.

(2) **Parkinson's Disease** — This disease is caused by the loss of neurons that synthesize a neurotransmitter called dopamine. Most of these neurons are located in a small area of the brain (a few centimeters long), called the *substantia nigra*. For unknown reasons, neuronal cells in this area die, and as the number of cells in this region drops, the disease progresses. If adult neural stem cells or ES cells could be turned into cells that are identical to those dying cells, then they can replace them and thus stop, or even reverse this disease. Since the affected area of the brain in Parkinson's disease is relatively small, it might be relatively easy to treat — much easier than, for example, pathologies such as Alzheimer's disease, which causes damage to several large areas of the brain. Such an attempt to repair a damaged brain with ES cells has been undertaken using animal models, and the results are very encouraging. For example, using a mouse as a model, it has been demonstrated that degenerating dopamine neurons can be replaced using ES cells.[8] These results should pave the way for human clinical trials. However, progress of the follow ups has not been reported, although it has already been 10 years.

(3) **Skin and Hair Restoration** — Skin might look like a simple thing at first glance — just like a sheet of leather. It is, however, a complex organ consisting of different cell types — cells that keep tissue together and provide elasticity (fibroblasts), cells that isolate skin from the environment and provide a protective barrier (keratinocytes), cells that provide skin

color and protect against UV rays (melanocytes), and others. Skin also contains different types of glands, such as sweat glands and sebaceous glands. Finally, skin forms hair follicles — mini-organs that produce hair. Therefore, stem cells must have the ability to differentiate into several different cell types and form several mini skin-organs to restore actual skin. This might sound like a "mission impossible." Surprisingly, a few years ago, a group from Switzerland discovered multipotent hair follicle stem cells that can generate several skin facets. When transplanted into a mouse model, these cells participate in hair follicle renewal, promote hair growth, and contribute to the formation of skin parts such as sebaceous glands and epidermis. Another group from the US claimed that stem cells implanted in a hairless mouse generated hair. This should be good news for bald people! Unfortunately, a few years later, no follow up progress has been made, and bald people still do not benefit from stem cells.

(4) **Diabetes** — There are several types of diabetes. One of its common forms, type 1, is caused by a loss of beta-cells in the pancreas, which secrete insulin. Regeneration of these cells could, theoretically, restore the production of insulin and cure diabetes. Unfortunately, how beta-cells are regenerated is not yet known. So far, researchers have not found any evidence of pancreatic adult stem cells, and probably only ES cells can be used to develop beta-cells. This looks feasible, but it might take some time.

(5) **Heart Failure** — Heart failure is one of the most common causes of death. It results from damage to the heart muscle, such as that which occurs after a heart attack. It leads to the heart's inability to pump enough blood to meet the body's needs. Several sources of stem cells have been tested to restore such damaged tissue, among them: bone marrow, cells from cell lines cultured in laboratories, and others. Unfortunately, the results have been poor so far, and the "recipe" for heart restoration has yet to be found. Nevertheless, in some cases the experiments were found to be beneficial, leading researchers to believe that stem cell therapy will be commonly used to restore heart tissue within the next 10 years.

(6) **Alzheimer's Disease** — It is unclear where the idea of treating of Alzheimer's disease using stem cells first came from. Probably, it began as a dream to treat such a common and devastating human disease, and then

traveled from publication to publication with little professional analysis. Such things do happen in science from time to time. But it seems that this disorder should be one of the last on the list of possible stem cell therapeutic targets. The problem is that Alzheimer's disease affects many brain regions, and almost half of the human brain in total. Specifically, it is caused by degeneration in the temporal lobe, parietal lobe, hippocampus, frontal cerebral cortex, and other parts of the brain. Treatment of this disease would therefore require regeneration of different types of neurons in extensive areas of the human brain. If one can learn how to re-grow half of the human brain, one probably can re-grow anything!

(7) **Toxicology and Drug Discovery** — This sounds like the least exciting application, but it is in fact the most likely immediate application of stem cells. Cells grown in dishes, flasks or tubes can be used to test new chemicals and drugs in screening for their targets and in evaluating their toxicity. So far, investigators have used two kinds of cells: (i) primary cells, which are isolated from adult tissues, and (ii) cell lines, which usually originate from tumors. The drawback of using tumor cells is that they are genetically abnormal and, therefore, they are not the best model for the evaluation of efficacy and toxicity. On the other hand, primary cells, which are perfectly normal, can divide only a limited number of times and do not survive in dishes for a long time. They can still be made to divide an unlimited number of times through a technique called immortalization. Immortalized cells, however, similarly to cancerous cells, are abnormal. Stem cells have neither of these disadvantages — they can divide and survive for a long time, and they are genetically normal cells. Thus, stem cells are a better model for the drug discovery process, and they can replace, at least partially, the need for both animal models and human testing. This would save a lot of time and money, and it would accelerate the drug discovery process in general.

Controversies

Probably no other technology currently raises more controversies than ES cell research. The opposition to this new research is based on moral, ethical, and religious grounds. The main question is — is one depriving ES cells of the potential to develop into complete human beings? The answer to this question depends on how one views the origin of human life — does it begin with the merging of a female egg with a male spermatozoid, or does it start sometime later? According to Jewish belief, human life starts only 40 days after conception. According to Muslim traditions, human life begins at the end of four months of pregnancy. Roman Catholic tradition is more conservative, and it suggests that human life begins at conception. Therefore, the Roman Catholic Church opposes ES cell research, while Muslim and Jewish traditions do not.

According to their cultural traditions and beliefs, various countries have applied different regulations on ES cell research. For example, French law permits the use of ES cells that are not needed (and most likely would be disposed of) by the genetic parents. US law does not permit the use of any ES cells, except for cells that existed before the law was introduced. Overall, however, countries that represent about 3.5 billion people (more than half the world's population) either completely permit use of ES cells or permit their use with some limitations.

The question of when human life actually starts depends on a person's religious, cultural, and philosophical views. It is recommended, dear reader, that you again take a look again at Fig. 4.3, which explains where ES cells come from, and make up your own mind — is someone killed to develop ES cells? Even if it is accepted that using the ES cells is unethical and immoral, the question still remains of what to do with those frozen embryos that have already been created for infertile families. It is estimated that there are around 400,000 such frozen embryos in the US alone, and it is unknown how many embryos are disposed of at clinics, after the parents have the babies they want and have approved their destruction. And what will happen to those 400,000 embryos sitting in the freezers? Likely, most of them will never be claimed. So it raises the question: Is it more ethical and moral to use them for research instead of storing and eventually destroying them?

New approaches for ES cell isolation have been devised to eliminate the controversies. For example, scientists at the company Advanced Cell Technology have developed a method in which a single cell from a developing embryo is isolated to create a cell line without destroying the embryo.[9] In a different approach, several publications in 2007 demonstrated that normal adult cells can be reprogrammed back to an embryonic state.[10] Moreover, it appears possible to create pluripotent cells, which are very similar to ES cells, from somatic adult cells (see above). There is only one difference between pluripotent and ES cells — pluripotent cells can differentiate into any cell type except for the embryonic type, whereas ES cells, which are called totipotent, can differentiate into any cell type including the embryonic type. Since pluripotent cells can differentiate into any cell type except for embryonic, they can be used to regenerate any tissue/organ, without the controversies associated with ES cells. By now, many successful approaches to create pluripotent cells have been reported: from mouse fibroblast (skin) cells in 2006,[2] from human fibroblast (skin) cells in 2007,[3,4] and from human spermatogonial (testis) cells in 2008,[6] followed by others. All these approaches help to solve the issue of killing a potential life, and it is very likely that other, new ways of ES cell isolation and ways of replacing ES cells with induced pluripotent cells (iPS) will be developed in the near future.

Future

Exciting prospects continue to reveal themselves as scientists discover new sources of stem cells. For example, blood stem cells can be isolated from a baby's umbilical cord. In 2007, a group of scientists from the US discovered another very potent stem cell source — the amniotic fluid which surrounds a developing embryo.[11] Even the Roman Catholic Church, which forbids the use of ES cells, has welcomed this news and, in 2010, called amniotic stem cells "the future of medicine." If samples of amniotic fluid and umbilical cords are preserved and saved from each baby, they can later be used to repair tissues or organs. Then, each individual can have a stored, perfectly matching source of stem cells. Banks with umbilical cord samples are already being created. These umbilical cord blood stem cell banks have already been successful in facilitating the treatment of individuals with certain hematological disorders and certain inherited metabolic diseases, such as Krabbe disease.

As shown above, stem cell technology has proved to not be as simple as it was originally hoped. The hope was that stem cells would somehow figure out how to differentiate and repair organs when implanted into damaged sites. As learned from the attempts to repair spinal cords, to restore hair, and to cure Parkinson's disease — stem cells do not work this way, but rather must be instructed on how to repair tissues or organs. Stem cells constantly receive chemical and physical signals that tell them what to do. When these signals are discovered and understood, we will know how to command cells to do what we want.

It seems that adult stem cells can be as multipotent as ES cells, so they might be the subject of choice in the future. Moreover, it is quite possible that all cells in the body are multipotent, and that sometime in the future, we might be able to use any type of cell to repair or regenerate our bodies, not only stem cells. Why is this possible? Because every cell of each particular individual contains identical DNA molecules that carry the human genome. Therefore, all human cells have identical genes. The trick is that our cells express only part of these genes at any given moment, and different types of cells express different sets of genes. How are the genes turned on or off? By physical or chemical signals. And if these signals are known, we could command one type of cell to behave as another type. For example, a neuron might be commanded to express the same set of genes as a muscle cell, and it might be transformed into a muscle cell.

Experiments with plants confirm such possibilities. Whole plants can be regenerated from any single cell — from a root cell, a leaf cell, etc. This means that somatic cells in plants are totipotent and, potentially, are stem cells. Tobacco plants, for example, have long been routinely regenerated from leaves under laboratory conditions. It took some time of course, to learn how to do this — to identify the nutrients and hormones for incubating cells, the temperature and characteristics of light to apply, etc. As of today, it has been learned how to regenerate dozens of different kinds of plants from different types of somatic cells. All plants are divided into two groups — monocots and dicots. Interestingly, until the 1990s only plants belonging to the group called dicots could be regenerated. No matter how hard scientists tried, they could not regenerate plants from the second group — monocot plants. This was quite a disappointment, because most of the important crops belong to this group, such as rice and wheat. The situation became so frustrating that some scientists proposed that cells of monocot plants were not totipotent, and that it was impossible to regenerate a whole plant from somatic cells from these kinds of plants. Guess what? A few years later, a whole rice plant, which belongs to monocots, was regenerated!

Indeed, as this book was almost ready to be published, scientists demonstrated that iPS cells originated from human skin can generate egg and sperm cells,[12] which then can be used to create embryos. Thus, these latest developments show that somatic cells have the potential to form embryos, which indicates that all cells in the body can be totipotent and leads to endless possibilities for stem cell technology in medicine.

References

1. Thomson JA, *et al.* (1998) Embryonic stem cell lines derived from human blastocysts. *Science* **282:** 1145–7.
2. Takahashi K, Yamanaka S. (2006) Induction of pluripotent stem cells from mouse embryonic and adult fibroblast cultures by defined factors. *Cell* **126:** 663–76.
3. Takahashi K, *et al.* (2007) Induction of pluripotent stem cells from adult human fibroblasts by defined factors. *Cell* **131:** 861–72.
4. Yu J, *et al.* (2007) Induced pluripotent stem cell lines derived from human somatic cells. *Science* **318:** 1917–20.
5. Vierbuchen T, *et al.* (2010) Direct conversion of fibroblasts to functional neurons by defined factors. *Nature* **463:** 1035–41.
6. Conrad S, *et al.* (2008) Generation of pluripotent stem cells from adult human testis. *Nature* **456:** 344–9.
7. Pollack A. (2011) Geron Is Shutting Down Its Stem Cell Clinical Trial. *The New York Times,* Nov 14, 2011.
8. Kim JH, *et al.* (2002) Dopamine neurons derived from embryonic stem cells function in an animal model of Parkinson's disease. *Nature* **418:** 50–6.
9. Chung Y, *et al.* (2008) Human embryonic stem cell lines generated without embryo destruction. *Cell Stem Cell* **2:** 113–7.

10. Cyranoski D. (2007) Simple switch turns cells embryonic. *Nature* **447:** 618–9.

11. De Coppi P, *et al.* (2007) Isolation of amniotic stem cell lines with potential for therapy. *Nat Biotechnol* **25:** 100–6.

12. Irie N, *et al.* (2014) SOX17 is a Critical Specifier of Human Primordial Germ Cell Fate. *Cell* **160:** 1–16.

CHAPTER 5

Nanomedicine

Definition

Nanotechnology can improve other technologies, including medical technology, information technology, communication technology and others. It is an interdisciplinary technology, which is difficult to define. Nevertheless, the terms nanotechnology and nanomedicine are widely used, and as such, will be explained in the best way possible.

Nanomedicine is the medical application of nanotechnology. Nanotechnology means literally "the technology of the small." How small? In the range of a nanometer; the prefix "nano" means one billion times smaller than one, meaning that one nanometer is 1,000,000,000 times smaller than one meter. Mathematically, a nanometer is expressed as 10^{-9} meter. It is accepted that nanotechnology deals with objects, materials, or devices that have one or more critical dimensions between 0.1 and 100 nanometers. For comparison, one nanometer is 80,000 times smaller than the diameter of a human hair! It is much smaller than any cell in the body (human cells generally have a diameter of between 10,000 and 20,000 nanometers). It is as small as some bio-molecules, such as the molecules of proteins. DNA molecules, from which genes are built, have a diameter in the range of 2.5 nanometers. Therefore, nanotechnology is a technology that allows the building of things with molecular precision. Building things at even smaller levels is also possible to imaging. In the future, it may be possible to manipulate atoms from which molecules are built, or even to manipulate sub-atomic and quantum elements. However, atomic and sub-atomic elements are considerably smaller than 0.1 nanometer; therefore, by current definition, manipulations at these levels cannot be included under the heading of nanotechnology. Some propose calling this quantum nanotechnology, or "nanotechnology of the next generation."

Overall, nanotechnology can be defined as the technology that allows the creation and use of systems, devices, and materials with new properties, resulting from their nanoscale size. Some also include in this definition the ability to understand these systems and materials. Understanding things on the nanoscale (and even smaller levels) began a very long time ago, in 1811, when the Italian chemist Avogadro first introduced the concept of molecules. Thus, according to the definition that includes "understanding," nanotechnology has already existed for over 200 years. In addition, according to this definition, any science that operates at molecular or lower levels could be classified as nanotechnology. This would be confusing, however, because most modern scientific disciplines (molecular biology, molecular physics, chemistry, etc.) operate at nanoscale levels.

As technology develops in the direction of smaller, more compact, and miniature scales, nanotechnology is poised to grow into a huge business. For example, it has been estimated that nanomedicine sales already reached $6.8 billion in the year 2004,[1] and a minimum of $3.8 billion is invested every year in nanotechnology research and development. Nanotechnology is a multidisciplinary technology which emerges from biological, chemical, physical, and engineering sciences. Also, it is expected that nanotechnology will contribute to many other fields of science. It is expected that it will further miniaturize computers and electronics. It is hoped that nanotechnology will help develop new environmentally friendly products. It is also to be expected that nanotechnology will contribute to the development of new materials and devices which will revolutionize energy technology, nutrition, transport technology, and military science. Nanotechnology will also have a huge impact on medicine. These medical applications, defined as "nanomedicine," will be examined here.

History

Although the actual term "nanotechnology" was first used by the Japanese engineer Taniguchi in 1974, the possibility of building small things was envisioned long before. In 1959, the famous American physicist Richard Feynman expressed the idea of building things at atomic levels. In one of his speeches he envisioned: "The principles of physics, as far as I can see, do not speak against the possibility of maneuvering things atom by atom." This may be easily said, but is very difficult to do. It was not until several years ago that manufacturing things at such small levels was considered viable. The ability to manipulate at nano-scale levels has largely been acce-lerated by recent advances in microscopy technology, such as the development of electron microscopy, atomic force microscopy, and scanning tunneling microscopy. Scanning tunneling microscopes, invented in the early 1980s by Swiss scientists, became an especially important contribution to nanotechnology. They allow such high-resolutions images that individual atoms become visible. Moreover, these instruments made it possible to relocate individual molecules and atoms. This opened up prospects for building materials and structures atom by atom, a process called the "bottom-up" approach.

Talking specifically about medical applications in nanotechnology, an important development came in 1991, when Sumio Iijima discovered a new form of carbon, the nanotube (see below for more details). As for now, businesses and governments alike consider nanotechnology to be the future of technology. Government-funded research programs have been launched in many industrialized countries. For example, in 2000, the US government created the billion-dollar National Nanotechnology Initiative. Similar programs were also launched by the EU Commission soon after. Research activities and initiatives have been increasing over the past several years, mostly at universities. Private businesses have also finally seen the opportunities, and commercial endeavors are now beginning to emerge.

Principles

Many materials show an interesting phenomenon: At the nano-scale, their properties differ drastically from the properties of large-sized bulk matter. These special properties are due to the fact that the ratio of sur-face-to-volume is higher in small quantities of matter than in large ones. Many chemical reactions take place on the surface of materials, and as the ratio of the surface to the volume increases, the material becomes more reactive. For example, fine particles of iron are flammable, while bulk iron is fire resistant. This phenomenon allows for the creation of materials with new properties and can make things stronger, less expensive, cleaner, etc. Nanotechnology has already found its practical applications, and many products using the unique properties of nano-scale materials are already used in everyday life: car bumper coatings, stain-free coatings, dental-bonding agents, metal-cutting tools, sunscreens, cosmetics, and others.

Nanotechnology is a technology emerging from several sciences, including biology, and it is hard to draw a border around them, especially between molecular biology and nanotechnology. It seems, however, that the use of bio-molecules naturally found in the body, without the application of artificial materials, should be considered molecular biology, rather than nanotechnology. For example, the isolation and use of genes for therapeutic purposes is not considered nanotechnology, but rather gene therapy, despite the fact that genes have nano-scale dimensions. Therefore, the principles of nanotechnology should include man-made things that are not naturally found in the body. Below are several examples of such things:

(1) **Nanotubes** — Carbon nanotubes are an icon of modern nanomedicine. Carbon can be found in two forms — pure carbon and graphite/diamond form. In 1991, the Japanese researcher Iijima discovered a third form of carbon — nanotube carbon. As the name suggests, atoms of this form of carbon are rolled up into tubes (Fig. 5.1). The walls of the tubes can be built from one or several layers of carbon atoms, and are only a few nanometers in diameter. The tubes, however, can be very long, reaching up to several centimeters (millions of nanometers). They are flexible and extremely strong.

Nanotubes can also be created using inorganic compounds, such as titanium dioxide, tungsten disulfide, and others. Nanotubes from these compounds can be even smaller than carbon nanotubes, and their diameter can be as small as a few tens of nanometers.

(2) **Nanofibers** — Nanofibers are made of natural or synthetic organic polymers, such as collagen, polyurethane, etc. They are very thin and have remarkable physical properties. Nanofibers can be inserted into cells without significantly damaging them or affecting their viability,

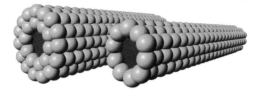

Figure 5.1. Carbon nanotubes. Atoms of carbon are rolled up into tubes. (Left) The tube is built from two layers of carbon atoms; (right) the tube is built from one layer of carbon atoms.

which makes them a promising tool for the controlled delivery of materials into cells. For example, genetic material (DNA) could be attached to nanofibers and delivered into cells in a controlled manner.

(3) **Nanowires** — In contrast to nanofibers, nanowires are made of inorganic materials, such as silicon, indium phosphide, and many others. They have unique electrical and optical properties.

(4) **Nanopores** — Nanopores are small holes that allow for the precise control of molecules passing through materials. They can be made of proteins, lipids, or nanotubes. In solid materials, nanopores can be made simply as very small holes.

(5) **Nanoparticles** — These are bulk particles that have a size of less than 100 nm. Nanoparticles can be made of many chemicals, including iron oxide, titanium oxide, colloidal gold, and others. They can be used either as suspensions, or attached to other materials. Nanoparticles are already widely used. Iron oxide nanocrystals, for example, possess supermagnetic properties and are used as contrast agents in magnetic resonance imaging (MRI). Forms of nanoparticles that consist of carbon atoms and create onion-like structures are called fullerenes. Nanoparticles made of semiconductor materials that adopt the form of crystals are called quantum dots.

(6) **Quantum Dots** — Quantum dots are very small particles, and their diameters can be only a few tenths of a nanometer. They are made of semiconductor materials and adopt the form of crystals. Because of their small size, the electrons that they contain begin to behave more like quantums, rather than particles. Quantum dots exchange energy

only at certain levels, and they absorb or emit only specific wavelengths of light. The emitted wavelength of light, and thus the color, can be changed by altering the quantum dots' size, making quantum dots suitable for labeling in many applications of molecular biology.

(7) **Nanolayers** — These are films or layers that are as little as one atom or one molecule thick. Nanolayers are used as coatings for various applications. For example, they are used to make bumpers on cars more resistant to damage.

(8) **Nanocarriers** — These are nanoscale materials that can be used either for the delivery of drugs that are hard to absorb by the body, or for the controlled release of drugs inside the body. For example, nanoparticles called dendrimers can be used as such vehicles. Dendrimers can self-assemble from smaller molecules to form branched shape structures, between which drugs can be attached.

Another example is the pH-responsive carriers, which are made of polymers sensitive to pH levels (degree of acidity) and able to destabilize cell membranes. These properties make them a promising tool for the delivery of drugs inside cells (Fig. 5.2). These polymers only become active once they penetrate inside cells and are released into the endosomal compartment. In endosomes, the polymer is exposed to a low pH level (high acidity) and separates from the drug to which

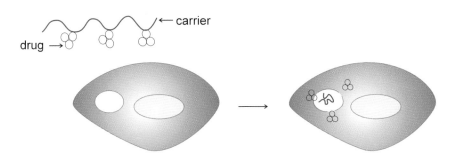

Fig. 5.2   Drug delivery using a pH-responsive carrier. A drug is attached to the carrier. The carrier is made of a polymer that is sensitive to pH and has the ability to destabilize cell membranes. It penetrates inside cells into the endosomal compartment (white circle). In the endosomes, the polymer is exposed to low pH (high acidity), causing it to separate from the drug to which it was attached. Next, the polymer destabilizes the endosomal membrane and allows the drug to leak inside the cell.

it was attached. Next, the polymer destabilizes the endosomal membrane, allowing the drug to leak out inside the cell.

Besides responses to pH, carriers that respond to magnetic fields, heat, or other physical stimuli are being developed. By controlling particles that carry a drug, one can control drug delivery rates into the body, as well as control the precise locations of the drug's release. This could revolutionize the pharmaceutical industry, and nanoscale-based delivery strategies have already begun to make an impact on pharmaceutical planning.

Technical Problems

Nanosystems, nanodevices, nanoparticles, and other nano-things (for simplicity, they will collectively be referred to as "nano-things") can dramatically enhance the ability to treat, monitor, and cure diseases. Unfortunately, when internalized, all those nano-things can be seen by the body as foreign particles that must be eliminated. The behavior of the nano-things within the body, their stability, their distribution through the body, and finally, their clearance and elimination from the body, depend upon several characteristics of the nano-things, such as their size, morphology (shape), and chemical makeup.

The liver and spleen perform the first step of clearing foreign objects from the body. Foreign things that are cleared by these two organs are further recognized and eliminated by the immune system. Therefore, in order to work with nano-things, one has to design them in such a way that one is able to predict and control their behavior inside the body. For example, they have to be designed to avoid their aggregation, which would inactivate them. One must also prevent their recognition by immune system cells, such as macrophage cells, which would eliminate them. These issues are still not sufficiently examined, and their understanding is necessary for the future progress of nanomedicine.

In addition, the knowledge of mechanisms of elimination of nano-things from the body can be exploited for their delivery into specific sites. For instance, since macrophages are concentrated by the sites of infections, the design of nano-things that will target macrophages can be used to deliver drugs to infection sites. Since a drug in this case will not be evenly spread throughout the body, but rather will be concentrated at specific sites, less of the drug will be required for the treatment. This would be of benefit economically, and also reduce the chances of side effects.

Macrophages are specialized host defense cells that engulf and digest cellular debris, as well as pathogens. In addition to the engulfing and digestion of foreign bodies, macrophages send specific signals that regulate the immune system. Therefore, macrophages can also be an appropriate target for the regulation of immunogenicity. In some disorders, such as autoimmune blood disorders, rheumatoid arthritis, and others, macrophages attack host (our own) cells, and they are harmful. Therefore, to treat such disorders, drugs that would inactivate macrophages should be designed in such manner that they would be specifically engulfed by macrophages, but not other cells.

Although nano-things can be very helpful in diagnosing and treating diseases, they in and of themselves could have toxic effects, or could even cause diseases. For example, it has been shown that fine particles can cause human lung cancer. Another example is carbon nanotubes, which can cause oxidative stress and cell death. Moreover, it has been demonstrated in experiments with animals that carbon nanotubes can be spread by blood into the lungs where they cause damage. Another form of carbon, known as "buckyballs" (which might enable faster speeds of internet and other data cables), has been shown to kill bacteria and brain cells in a fish model. Therefore, the fate and effects of nano-things must be carefully examined before their application on humans, and before their release into the environment.

Applications

In medicine, nanotechnology can have a wide range of applications. It can be used to diagnose, treat, and monitor diseases. In order to do so, one must be able to perform several things: (1) identify specific markers of particular diseases or medical conditions — in other words, one has to be able to recognize a disease or a medical condition; (2) figure out what physical procedures or drugs can specifically treat the disease, with minimal side effects; (3) figure out how to deliver such physical procedures or drugs, in the most efficient way and with minimal side effects. For example, someone with a brain tumor — to cure this person, first, the tumor must be recognized, and then it must be determined exactly what kind of tumor it is. Second, the proper irradiation or drugs that will specifically kill the tumor cells but leave all other cells unaffected must be found. Third, we have to be able to deliver the irradiation or a drug into the tumor, inside the brain, without harming normal tissues and organs. If the tumor is misdiagnosed, the wrong procedure or the wrong drug could be used, and would not kill the tumor cells. If a drug that does not penetrate the blood–brain barrier is injected, the drug will not be delivered, and it will not kill the tumor cells, etc. Nanotechnology can be very useful for solving these problems with minimal side effects.

(1) **Cancers** — Nanotechnology offers very promising tools to fight cancers. First, it can improve our ability for early detection, which makes it easier to treat them. Second, it can enhance our ability to kill cancer cells with minimal side effects.

The application of nanotechnology in molecular imaging already allows for the enhanced detection of tumors. The goal of the imaging is to detect tumor masses that have 1,000 cells or fewer, as opposed to current techniques, which usually detect tumors that have 1,000,000 cells or more. Indeed, nanotechnology has already improved the detection of metastases in lymph nodes in patients with prostate cancer. Using a new approach that utilizes paramagnetic iron oxide crystals, metastases that measure less than 2 mm in diameter can be detected. Similar supermagnetic nanoconstructs have also been successfully used for the detection of pathologies associated with arthritis and other diseases.

When it comes to eliminating tumors, nanotechnology approaches are also already used. Examples include the drug Doxil, developed to treat AIDS-related Kaposi's sarcoma, as well as the drug Abraxane, which is used in the treatment of breast cancer. These drugs both employ nanocarriers. Doxil is doxorubicin placed into a capsule (liposome) made of polyethylene glycol. Abraxane is paclitaxel bonded to albumin as a delivery vehicle. Both of these drugs have already been used in clinical practice for several years. Moreover, other carriers that target cancer cells more selectively are currently being tested. Scientists from Washington University, St. Louis, in the US, successfully created the so-called "nanobees" — nanoparticles made of perfluorocarbon, in which the toxin from bee venom is incorporated.[2] Perfluorocarbon is an inert material used in artificial blood. Nanoparticles made of it are small enough to pass through the bloodstream and attach to cells, yet large enough to carry a number of drugs. When administered in the body, nanobees accumulate in the tumors, because tumors have leaky blood vessels and tend to retain materials. Then, the bee toxin contained in nanoparticles, mellitin, can be released and "drill" holes in cancer cells, destroying them without any apparent signs of toxicity to the rest of the body. However, these nanobees have only been tested on mice so far.

Besides nanocarriers, other techniques to fight cancers are also being tested. A very promising technique employing carbon nanotubes has recently been developed by several research teams in the US. A team from the California Institute of Technology has demonstrated that single-walled carbon nanotubes can be used to kill cancer cells.[3] The nanotubes can be bound to agents that specifically attach to cancer but not to normal cells. Then, the area of the tumor can be irradiated with an infrared laser that passes through normal cells without heating them, but that heats nanotubes attached to cancer cells, thus killing the cancer cells. This principle was developed earlier by another laboratory using gold nanoshells instead of carbon nanotubes.[4] This approach has also been modified to kill cells using chemicals, such as cisplatin, instead of high temperatures.[5] In the future, it would be very beneficial to identify and test specific molecules, such as antibodies, that target and bind to particular kinds of cancer cells. Several such cancer antibodies are already known, and it is possible that their use as an attachment for nanotubes will allow the creation of more specific and efficient anti-cancer treatments.

Cancer cells constantly grow and divide, and for this they need nutrients that come with blood. Therefore, growing cancers initiate the formation of new blood vessels that will feed them. This process is called angiogenesis. If we can shut down blood supply to tumors, we can stop their growth and kill them by "starvation." Such approaches have already been successfully tested. For example, researchers have been able to target growing blood vessels using quantum dots and liposomes that were coated with specific proteins.

(2) **Diagnostics and Imaging** — Nanomaterials can be used to visualize cells and tissues in the body. This allows for the detection of anatomical and physiological changes in the bodies, which helps in the detection and monitoring of diseases. To do this, nanomaterials are first labeled, then injected or swallowed, and made visible in the body using tomography, MRI, or optical methods. The labeling is usually done by attaching radioactive or contrast coloring agents to nanomaterials. The application of quantum dots instead of traditional radioactive or coloring agents for labeling is also possible; this method has been tested intensively over the last several years. Current techniques already achieve very fine resolutions and allow for the visualization of living cells in the body. For example, particles that combine dendrimers with supermagnetic nanoparticles of iron oxide have been successfully used to monitor the migration and division of transplanted cells in animal models. In the future, this could be very valuable for monitoring cells in tissues that were transplanted using stem cell therapy. In addition, labeling agents in and of themselves can sometimes act as a medicine. For example, when irradiated with laser light, some coloring/fluorescent agents produce toxic materials that kill cancer cells.

Nanowires have also been shown as a very promising tool. Sensor test chips containing nanowires have been demonstrated to be a selective and sensitive tool in the detection of proteins and other markers associated with cancers and other diseases.[6] Therefore, nanowires could enable the early detection and diagnosis of many human diseases.

(3) **Identification and Monitoring** — Small chips with attached radio antennas can be used for labeling many materials. Such labels are called RFID (radio frequency identification) labels. In these devices, a chip is used to store information, and an antenna transmits it. RFID labels are already used for many purposes in medical practices. For example, they are used to "label" newborn babies or demented patients, to prevent their abduction or their getting lost. They are also used to label and trace medicines or medical equipment. In 2004, such devices, which have the size of a grain of rice, were approved in the US to store a person's medical

records. This device can be implanted under the skin and used in emergency cases to retrieve a patient's medical information, which can be vital for treatment and even save a patient's life. Further miniaturization of such devices will make them even more valuable in the future.

Nanotechnology has recently contributed to amazing progress in the manufacturing of devices that monitor blood glucose in diabetics. These devices, based on implantable platinum electrodes, carry glucose sensors to continuously monitor glucose levels. The electrodes can be placed just under the skin and will measure glucose levels every five minutes. The results are then transmitted to a wireless hand-held device that shows graphic information, provides alerts for low or high blood sugar, etc. Such a device is already in widespread clinical use, manufactured by Dexcom, Inc., located in the US.

(4) **Drug Delivery** — Currently, drugs are either directly injected into tissues or swallowed. This method of drug delivery has several potential problems: (i) not all drugs can be dissolved in tissues or blood; (ii) some drugs cannot pass barriers within the body, such as placenta and the blood–brain barrier (thus, making them unable to reach the treatment site); (iii) when absorbed, drugs are distributed randomly throughout the body, accumulating not only in diseased tissues, but also in healthy tissues, causing side effects; (iv) many drugs are broken down and inactivated in the body before they reach the diseased tissues. All of this contributes to a reduction in drug bioavailability and huge resources (more than $65 billion) are wasted each year due to this issue. Nanotechnology can help overcome these problems. Drugs can be attached to or encapsulated in nanocarriers, such as dendrimers (see above) that are designed to deliver and release them to the right place in the body. For example, such a delivery system is already in use for the treatment of visceral leishmaniasis, and also against some fungal infections using a drug called amphotericin B. In this system, the drug is encapsulated in nanoparticles that are built from lipids. Another good example is the drug abraxane, which is approved for treating breast cancer. This drug basically represents paclitaxel bound to the nanoparticle albumin, and has been shown to be significantly more efficient in comparison to standard paclitaxel.[7] More

nanocarriers that deliver drugs to site-specific locations and release them at set rates are currently under development.

(5) **Disinfection** — The disinfectant properties of some chemicals, such as silver, have been known for a long time. Using them as nanoparticles makes the chemicals even more potent bacteria killers. Several chemicals are already used for disinfection, among them silver, titanium dioxide, and others. Nanocrystalline silver, for example, is currently used for antimicrobial wound dressings. As the problem of bacterial resistance to antibiotics becomes more frequent, using such nanomaterials becomes especially important as an additional way to kill bacteria. They are even more attractive because the mechanisms by which these chemicals kill bacteria are multiple, and bacteria are unlikely to become resistant to them.

(6) **Repair of Tissues** — Artificial bone joints are currently one of the most useful applications of nanotechnology for tissue repair. The material at bone joints wears off relatively fast, and the lifetime of artificial joints made from conventional materials is usually not more than 15 years. One of the most promising uses of nanomaterials currently is hydroxyapatite. This material resembles the natural material of bones. It consists of 70% hydroxyapatite mineral and 30% of organic fibers made from collagen. Although this material has been used as a coating for implants for some time, modern technology has made it possible to apply the material in nanometer layers, as opposed to the micrometer layers used before. This makes the artificial joint more like natural bone, in which hydroxyapatite grains have a size of less than 50 nm. Such layers are more compatible with natural bones, and can even stimulate the growth and repair of surrounding tissues. Other materials, such as metal-ceramic and diamond, are also currently being tested for use as implant coatings.

Cells receive signals from the outside, and their behavior depends on these signals. In other words, cell-to-cell interaction and cell environment are important factors in the formation of tissue. Nanomaterials can be used to imitate an appropriate environment for cells, and thus to direct them to form specific tissues. Promising results have been achieved using nanofibers to regenerate brain tissue by a group of scientists from the US and

China.[8] In their experiments, researchers blinded hamsters by damaging specific areas of the brain. Next, they injected the hamsters with peptides (building blocks of proteins) that can self-assemble into nanofibers. After nanofibers were self-assembled, they were able to heal the brain and to restore the vision in the animals. Thus, this technology opens up the possibility of repairing damaged human nerves.

(7) **Neural Prostheses** — These devices are intended to restore or to take over nerve functions. Such prostheses already exist and are widely used. For example, pacemakers for regulating the heartbeat, cochlear implants for restoring hearing, and brain stimulators to reduce tremors associated with Parkinson's disease, among others. Current prostheses, however, are made using micro-level technologies, and building them at smaller (nano) levels would improve them dramatically.

A great deal of research is now being conducted to develop "artificial retinas," which could be implanted to restore vision in patients with damaged retinas. Researchers are trying to replace the damaged retinas with electrodes (see more details in Chapter 7). They have now developed electrodes with nanoporous surfaces, significantly improving signal transfers from the electrodes to the tissue.

Very exciting research is now being conducted to develop neuroprostheses that can be operated by thought. To do this, chips with electrodes are connected to the area of the brain that registers the electrical signals associated with thoughts. The chips then receive signals from the brain, analyze them, and send appropriate signals to the organs. The first of such chips, which are also called brain-controlled interfaces, have already been created and successfully used in monkeys to operate both a robot arm and the cursor of a computer (review Ref. 9). Over the past few years, several groups of scientists have reported neuroprostheses that restored functions in a paralyzed man. In these experiments, the prosthesis enabled the man to perform several tasks using his thoughts: operating a light switch, selecting television channels, operating the cursor of a computer, and even playing video games. However, our understanding of the human brain is still too far away from being truly comprehensive, so it will likely be many more years before brain-controlled interfaces are used in medical practice.

Controversies

Although very new, nanomedicine already raises controversies. As this technology develops further, the amount of controversy will probably increase.

(1) **Doctor–Patient Relationship** — Nanotechnology will increase the number of devices available to detect, monitor, and treat conditions in the home environment. As a result, some procedures that are currently carried out by medical specialists will instead be performed at home, without them. However, it is not currently clear how far such processes can go without the presence of specialists. For example, there are no concerns when patients perform at home procedures such as monitoring their temperature or blood pressure. But there are concerns when patients perform self-diagnoses for pregnancy, HIV status, or such severe diseases as breast cancer. Devices that allow performing such tasks are already on the market, and some of them can be purchased through the internet. Many of these nanotech procedures, however, could involve enormous psychological consequences, and may require the presence of specialists.

(2) **Human Enhancement** — Although enhancements like connecting the human brain to a computer or the creation of cyborgs are in the distant future, some enhancements of humans can already be accomplished now. For example, artificial retinas to restore the sight of blind people are already a reality. Such retinas, theoretically, can also be used to enable people to see infrared radiation, which would give people the ability to see in the dark. Another example is cochlear implants, which could enable hearing at levels that the normal human ear cannot hear. Such enhancements raise moral questions — should they be performed at all, and if yes, who should get them? Performing these kinds of human enhancements would change human culture and even humans as a biological species.

(3) **Privacy** — Nanotechnology will facilitate data processing, storage and distribution. The whole medical history of a patient can be stored in small chips. This, however, makes it easier for unauthorized people to obtain information. If RFID is used, private information could be intercepted and stolen, similar to the interception of telephone conversations.

(4) **Fair Distribution** — Nanomedicine is a sophisticated technology, and as such, it is expensive. Therefore, there is concern that most of the improvements brought by nanomedicine will be available mostly to the richest, leading to concerns that nanotechnology might increase the division between poor and rich people. It might also widen the gap between developed and developing nations.

Future

It seems that the most immediate benefits of nanotechnology will be seen in the field of diagnostics. Medical instruments should become smaller, faster, and more precise. This means that smaller amounts of samples will be required to analyze conditions and diseases. Also, shorter times for analysis will be required. For example, smaller amounts of blood will be required for testing, and syringes would eventually be made at nanoscale sizes. Using such syringes, blood tests could be performed without compromising the skin and without the pain. Test results would be ready within hours, instead of the days that are required now.

In the more distant future, analyzing devices could be made as small as a single red blood cell, which has a diameter of about 8,000 nanometers. Making even smaller devices could become possible. Such devices will easily fit into the human circulatory system, and could even penetrate individual cells. Then, instead of taking samples of blood or tissues for analysis, miniature devices that monitor health could be implanted or injected into the body. They may be small RFID devices that can freely move throughout the circulatory systems and transmit information about our health to analyzing machines outside. Such devices would provide real-time information on biological processes taking place in the body. Even better would be coupling such devices with specific drugs to treat diseases. For example, it could be possible to create nanodevices measure blood-cholesterol levels and, at the same time, release anti-cholesterol drugs when they detect that cholesterol levels have become too high. This could also be done to detect and treat infections, toxic materials, or tumor cells.

It usually takes about 10 years to develop a new drug. This includes both time for development, as well as time for testing efficacy and safety. Nanodevices are no exception. There will need to be time for development, as well as time for testing. Therefore, it will take at least another 10 years before such new devices could appear in medical practice.

Also, such phenomena as self-assembly of functional structures from molecules or small particles might find a range of applications. This process, called "bottom-up manufacturing," would be especially useful for tissue repair. Such techniques are already being developed. For example, such bottom-up manufacturing was used to restore nerve function in the hamster model (see above, Repair of Tissues). This approach may also be useful in bone regeneration, wound closure, and nerve regeneration. Nanomedicine may even go beyond the repairing of tissue to its natural state. It might replace normal human tissues with ones that have new, advanced properties! Although this may sound like fantasy now, some think that such advances could become a reality within the next 20 years.

References

1. Freitas RA Jr. (2005) What is nanomedicine? *Nanomedicine* **1:** 2–9.
2. Soman NR, *et al.* (2009) Molecularly targeted nanocarriers deliver the cytolytic peptide melittin specifically to tumor cells in mice, reducing tumor growth. *J Clin Invest* **119:** 2830–42.
3. Kam NW, O'Connell M, Wisdom JA, Dai H. (2005) Carbon nanotubes as multifunctional biological transporters and near-infrared agents for selective cancer cell destruction. *Proc Natl Acad Sci USA* **102:** 11600–5.
4. Loo C, *et al.* (2004) Nanoshell-enabled photonics-based imaging and therapy of cancer. *Technol Cancer Res Treat* **3:** 33–40.
5. Dhar S, Liu Z, Thomale J, *et al.* (2008) Targeted single-wall carbon nanotube-mediated Pt(IV) prodrug delivery using folate as a homing device. *J Am Chem Soc* **130:** 11467–76.
6. Zheng G, Patolsky F, Cui Y, *et al.* (2005) Multiplexed electrical detection of cancer markers with nanowire sensor arrays. *Nat Biotechnol* **23:** 1294–301.
7. Gradishar WJ. (2005) Albumin-bound nanoparticle paclitaxel. *Clin Adv Hematol Oncol* **3:** 348–9.
8. Ellis-Behnke RG, *et al.* (2006) Nano neuro knitting: peptide nanofiber scaffold for brain repair and axon regeneration with functional return of vision. *Proc Natl Acad Sci USA* **103:** 5054–9.
9. Schwartz AB, Cui XT, Weber DJ, Moran DW. (2006) Brain-controlled interfaces: movement restoration with neural prosthetics. *Neuron* **52:** 205–20.

CHAPTER 6

Pharmacogenomics

Definition

Our environment and lifestyle can affect our response to medical treatment. Apparently, our genetic makeup also affects the body's response to medicines. Pharmacogenomics is the technology that analyzes how the genetic makeup of an individual affects his/her response to drugs. Pharmacogenomics is also called pharmacogenetics. As the word suggests, it combines the knowledge of pharmacology and of genetics (the knowledge of drugs and the knowledge of genes).

Each individual may respond differently to specific drugs. This is because, although the genomes of different people are similar, they are not identical, and each individual has a slightly different and unique genetic makeup. The differences in each individual's genetic makeup lead to the production of slightly different protein/enzyme profiles in each person. As a result, each person metabolizes drugs differently. In spite of this fact, the same drugs and the same doses are currently prescribed to different people to treat the same conditions. However, one size does not fit all! It is estimated that "one-formula-fits-all" drugs work for only 60% of the population, leaving at least 40% of patients at risk for adverse drug reactions. For example, certain prescription painkillers work well for some people, but not at all for others. Almost three million people in the US are at risk of overdose when prescribed standard amounts of common blood clot drugs alone. A change in just one single gene can be fatal for some patients treated with the standard dose of anti-leukemia drugs.

Overall, it is estimated that every year about 106,000 people die, and more than two million are hospitalized in the US alone as a result of adverse drug responses.[1] Ironically, this makes adverse drug reactions one of the leading causes of hospitalization and death.

History

The history of pharmacogenomics goes back to the 1950s, when researchers first noticed that responses to drugs can be inherited. For example, they noticed that the responses to specific drugs can vary based on race or ethnicity. It has been observed that responses to muscle relaxant drugs, anesthetics and other drugs often vary depending on the genetic background of patients. It has also been found that a small set of otherwise healthy people of certain genetic backgrounds can have fatal responses to inhaled anesthetics. The involvement of genetic factors in adverse drug reactions was first suggested in 1957 by Arno Motulsky.[2] At the same time, researchers identified enzyme deficiencies (caused by mutations in genes) that explained these adverse reactions to drugs. This allowed development of the concept of pharmocogenetics, which was first introduced in 1959 by German scientist Friedrich Vogel in his paper "Moderne Probleme der Humangenetik."[3] However, the crucial step in pharmaco-genomics was taken in the 1990s, when DNA single nucleotide polymorphisms (SNPs) were first discovered. SNPs (pronounced "snips") were found when scientists began sequencing DNA, which is built from four chemicals, called bases: adenine (A), guanine (G), cytosine (C), and thymine (T). These bases pair with their respective partners in order to create a double strand of DNA. Scientists noticed that, at some locations, DNA becomes polymorphic: One of the bases gets replaced with another, creating SNP (Fig. 6.1). More exactly, this happens once every 1,300 bases or so. Since the human genome consists of about three billion bases, it is estimated that the genome of each human has an average of 2.3 million SNPs.

It was also found that individual responses to drugs are oftentimes linked to specific patterns of SNPs. For example, the success of the hepatitis C virus treatment that employs a combination of interferon with ribavirin depends on SNPs (Fig. 6.1). Therefore, knowing an individual's

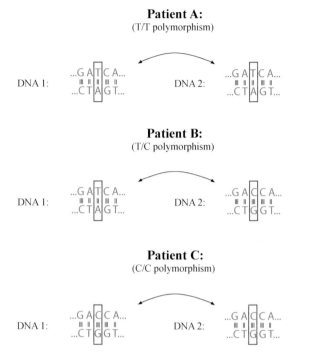

Fig. 6.1   Relationship between SNPs and the success of hepatitis C treatment. SNP that is found on chromosome 19 near the IL28B gene strongly affects the response of patients to hepatitis C treatment using interferon. SNPs are boxed.

Note: All somatic human cells are diploid, which means that they contain two sets of DNA (two alleles).

   Patient A: both DNAs of the patient contain T (T/T genotype). **Patient B:** one DNA of the patient contains C while another one contains T (C/T genotype). **Patient C:** both DNAs of the patient contain C (C/C genotype). It has been demonstrated that patients with C/C genotype are two to three times more likely to clear hepatitis C virus relative to the patients with the C/T or T/T genotypes.[4,5]

patterns of SNPs can help predict his/her response to drugs. In 1999, the SNP Consortium Ltd., made of pharmaceutical companies, bio-informational companies, academic research centers, and a charitable trust, began to identify and publish SNP maps. The consortium has now made publicly available maps of more than one million SNPs. Many pharmaceutical companies are also compiling their own collections, with the hope of using them in the development of new treatments. Large multinational consortia have also been established, such as the Electronic Medical Records and Genomics (eMERGE) Network, for storing such data in a Pharmacogenomics Knowledge Base.

Principles

Presently, pharmacogenomics is mostly based on associations between specific SNPs and the behavior of drugs in the body. SNPs are caused by changes in a single base of a DNA sequence (see Fig. 6.1). They represent one of the main factors behind genetic polymorphisms and variation between humans. How can SNPs affect drug behavior in the body? They modify genes, and modified genes produce modified proteins. In turn, the modification of proteins changes their interaction with drugs, such as their absorption into the body, the speed of drug breakdown (metabolism), drug interactions with target cells, conversion of drugs into more active or less active forms, and other interactions. Recently, however, it was found that non-coding (non-genic) DNA sequences can affect drug behavior in the body even more than the coding sequences. It appears that such sequences may produce a variety of RNAs that are not translated into proteins. In fact, recent studies prove that close to 30,000 genes make such strands of RNA, rather than proteins.[6] Depending on their size, these RNAs are called micro (miRNAs), small interfering RNA (siRNAs), or small RNAs. Although not translated into proteins, these RNAs can inter-act with and block RNAs that are translated into proteins, called mRNAs. SNPs in these non-coding RNAs can influence their ability to interact with mRNAs, affecting both their translation into proteins, as well as the body's interaction with drugs. It is estimated, for example, that miRNAs alone can block the translation of at least 30% of all genes. Surprising or not, currently known SNPs associated with diseases are found much more often in non-coding, compared to coding, DNA sequences.[7]

Before pharmacogenomics, the old-fashioned method of trial and error was used to figure out how the body interacts with medicines. Now, since certain patterns of SNPs have been shown to be linked to the body's inter-action with medicines (see Fig. 6.2), scientists can predict how drugs will work for each individual.

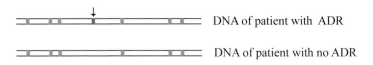

Fig. 6.2 Link between SNPs and drug effects. DNA strands are shown as horizontal lines. Vertical lines represent SNPs. Certain patterns of SNPs, as is indicated by the arrow, are associated with adverse drug reactions (ADR).

In order to know an individual's SNPs, his/her DNA has to be examined (sequenced). Sequencing of the whole genome, however, is currently a very slow and expensive process. Instead, DNA microarrays (DNA chips) are now being used. DNA chip technology is easy to automate, making it quick and affordable. A single chip can now be used to check about 100,000 SNPs in a patient's genome in a matter of several hours.

However, not all SNPs are associated with drug interactions or play a particular role in the behavior of drugs in the body. Some SNPs do not play any role, while some are very important. For example, SNPs located in cytochrome P450 genes are one of the most important indicators of the body's interaction with drugs. These genes encode enzymes, known as cytochromes P450 (CYP), which are produced in the liver. CYP enzymes are responsible for metabolizing approximately 80% of currently prescribed medicines.[8] Less active or inactive forms of CYP enzymes can cause the slow metabolism of drugs, which leads to their accumulation within the body to toxic levels, causing side effects. On the other hand, if the enzymes are too active, they can eliminate the drugs from the body so fast that the drugs have no chance of having a lasting therapeutic effect. Therefore, instead of analyzing the whole genome, one can gain a good idea of the body's interaction with most medicines by analyzing only those SNPs located in CYP genes. Today, such analyses are not yet performed in medical facilities. Nevertheless, SNP analyses are already frequently performed at research facilities and in medical trials.

Other important SNPs are found in the gene responsible for encoding the enzyme called dihydropyrimidine dehydrogenase. This enzyme is responsible for breaking down 5-fluorouracil (5-FU) — one of the most commonly used medicines in chemotherapy. Some polymorphisms in this gene cause deficiencies in the enzyme, leading to the accumulation of 5-FU in treated patients. High levels of 5-FU can be toxic and even lethal. Analyzing this gene sequence can predict who has such a deficiency, allowing doctors to adjust the dose of 5-FU in such cases in order to prevent adverse side effects from the drug.

SNPs in several other genes were shown to affect the rate of metabolism of other drugs used in chemotherapy. Knowing ahead of time who might have deficiencies in the enzymes encoded by these genes will help doctor adjust drug doses, and prevent dangerous adverse reactions during cancer treatment utilizing certain chemotherapies.

SNP genotyping is the most valuable tool in pharmacogenomics. However, other tools can also be used. Oftentimes, adverse drug effects can be caused by either excessive or insufficient gene expression. Therefore, some predictions about drug behavior in the body can be made by measuring the expression of certain genes. Gene expression measurement is usually done using DNA chips that measure levels of mRNA. Another way to evaluate gene expression is to measure the quantity of proteins encoded by genes. This can be done by using protein chips.

Technical Problems

The main challenge of pharmacogenomics is the complexity of finding gene variations that affect drug responses. First, a large number of SNPs has to be analyzed. As a result, pharmacogenomic testing is currently expensive. At this time, the cost of genotyping is about one dollar per SNP. Considering that each human has about 2.3 million SNPs, the cost for testing all SNPs would currently run around $2.3 million per patient! This is not practical, and in order to apply pharmacogenomics routinely in medical practice, the cost must go down. This could happen very soon due to recent advances in DNA sequencing technologies (see Future section below). Second, the SNPs cannot always clearly predict how each and every drug would behave in the body. Clear marker SNPs for the behavior of many drugs still remain to be found. It is estimated that about 8,000 genes can be drug targets, which opens up wide opportunities for finding new markers. As our knowledge about SNPs increases, more accurate predictions can, in theory, be made for more drugs. Currently, there is a race to catalog as many SNPs in the human genome as possible.

Another problem is limited drug alternatives and disincentives for pharmaceutical companies to produce multiple drugs. There may be only one or two drugs available for a certain condition, and if genomic variations in patients prevent them from using such drug(s), then they will be left with no alternative treatments.

Finally, pharmocogenomics will introduce an extra step to the drug prescription process. Physicians will have to learn how to accurately interpret the tests and choose the best treatment regimen for each patient. This will change the way doctors prescribe drugs in not just one field, but in all fields of medicine, and would require educating a large number of physicians concurrently.

Applications

Pharmacogenomics will allow for the prescription of better drug choices and for safer drug dosing. Before being approved for use, drugs must undergo rigorous testing, both for efficacy and safety. Although prescribed drugs are safe for most people, they can be toxic to other patients due to variations in their genes. Pharmacogenomics can predict who will have a negative effect from a drug, and who will respond well to a particular drug. Moreover, an effective drug dose can be predicted for each patient, based on his/her genetic makeup. This will help reduce the toxic side effects of drugs and increase their effectiveness, leading to lower patient mortality and morbidity, and lower cost of medical treatments. In the near future, pharmacogenomics will probably be the most valuable in such areas as oncology, psychiatry, and new drug development.

(1) **Oncology** — In many cancer treatments, the percentage of patients who respond well to treatments is low. This is especially true in chemotherapy, in which, very often, most patients do not respond to therapy as expected. Therefore, predictions of how a patient will react to drugs are especially needed in oncology. Such predictions have already been made for the anticancer drug called trastuzumab.

Trastuzumab is a genetically engineered antibody, used to treat metastatic breast cancer. It was developed by Genentech, and is sold under the name Herceptin. It has been shown that this medicine works well for only 25–30% of women, and those women who respond well overexpress one particular protein — the human epidermal growth factor receptor (HER2). Therefore, by measuring the HER2 levels in patients, one can predict who will respond to this drug. Although this is not a true pharmacogenomical test (it analyzes levels of a protein rather than the genetic makeup), this test is the first example demonstrating how pharmacogenomics can help in drug treatments.

Several other pharmocogenomical tests can now be performed to predict a patient's response to chemotherapy. Among them are tests that analyze variations in the dihydropyrimidine dehydrogenase gene and cytochrome P450 genes (see above, Principles). The US Food and Drug Administration (FDA) also recommends genetic testing before the treatment of acute lymphoblastic leukemia with the chemotherapy drug mercaptopurine (Purinethol). Pharmocogenomic testing is also now recommended before administering irinotecan (Camptosar), which is part of a combination chemotherapy regimen.

Another well known example regarding benefits of prescreening cancer patients for specific genetic alterations is the mutational status of the EGFR gene in non-small cell lung cancer (NSCLC), which is the most common type of lung cancer. Typically, this cancer is treated using either erlotinib or gefitinib. However, some patients respond to these drugs much better than others, depending on mutations in the EGFR gene. For example, NSCLC patients that have exon 19 deletions respond to the treatments much better.[9] On the other hand, patients that have exon 20 insertions have been associated with much lower response, which renders them unsuitable for therapies using either erlotinib or gefitinib.

Although pharmacogenomics can be extremely useful in cancer treatments, the relationship between genetic makeup of patients and their response to most of anticancer drugs is still far from known. This includes even the most widely used and life savings drugs such as imatinib. Imatinib, which is marketed by Novartis as Glivec, is one of the first molecularly targeted therapies. It has been proven efficient in treatment of a wide range of cancers, such as chronic myelogenous leukemia (CML), gastrointestinal stromal tumors and others. It is one of the most expensive drugs, costing a patient about $92,000 a year, with huge annual revenue of $4.7 billion in 2012. However, as with most drugs, imatinib causes toxic side effects in some patients while other patients develop resistance to it, and which genetic variations cause these problems still remains to be found.

(2) **Psychiatry** — For many drugs prescribed to patients with depression, beneficial effects are observed after only four to six weeks. If the drugs do not work, it results in a poor quality of life for the patient for a substantially long time. Therefore, the prediction of effects for this class of drugs would be very valuable. Such predictions can already be made for several drugs used in psychiatry. For example, it has been found that alterations in the CYP2D6 gene are associated with the rate of metabolism for the antidepressant called nortriptyline. Some variations in this gene cause ultra-rapid metabolism of nortriptyline and, as a result, the drug is eliminated from the body before exerting its healing effects. Such patients require higher drug doses, and the doctor could prescribe them if he/she knew ahead of time about alterations in his/her patient's CYP2D6 gene. Similar predictions can also be made for such drugs used in psychiatry and neurology as haloperidol, phenytoin, and others. Recently, genetic variations that affect the response of people with depression to citalopram (Celexa) were identified. This drug belongs to a widely used class of antidepressants called selective serotonin re-uptake inhibitors (SSRIs). Clinical trials are now underway to test whether pharmacogenomics can improve outcomes of SSRI treatment.

(3) **Drug Development** — Before new drugs are approved for sale, they have to be tested in clinical trials for safety and efficacy. Pharmaceutical companies have to test them on thousands of people, and it takes years to perform such trials. Companies spend an average of more than $250 million for each trial. However, if they knew ahead of time that people with certain genetic variations will not respond well to a drug or will have an adverse reaction, they could exclude such

people from clinical trials. This would reduce the number of patients required for a trial. As a result, the time and cost to develop a new drug would also be reduced. Pharmacogenomics may also revitalize some drugs that were previously abandoned during their development. For example, the development of bucindolol (Gencaro) was stopped some time ago because it did not show promise. However, recent tests found that this drug works well in patients with two genetic variants that regulate heart function, but does not work well with other patients. Thus, this drug can be efficient for certain patients and, if approved, Gencaro could become the first new drug that would require (not just have recommended) genetic testing before its prescription.

(4) **Others** — As described above, pharmacogenomics has been demonstrated to be very useful in hepatitis C treatment. As shown in Fig. 6.1, a polymorphism near a human interferon gene that is predictive for the effectiveness of interferon treatment for hepatitis C has been identified.[4,5] These studies demonstrated that patients with a certain genetic pattern near the IL28B gene are more responsive to the treatment than others. Therefore, knowing the IL28B genetic pattern can help in making decisions regarding hepatitis C treatment, and commercial tests for IL28B genotyping is already available in North America.

Interestingly, individuals can react very differently even to dietary supplements, such as vitamin E. Regarding patients with diabetes, it has been found that vitamin E provides cardiovascular protection to some, but harms others. Apparently, this depends on genetics too: It protects patients with the haptoglobin 2-2 genotype, but appears to harm patients with the haptoglobin 2-1 genotype.[10] Thus, pharmacogenetics should be applied to diabetic patients to make decisions regarding their cardiovascular health.

Controversies

Pharmacogenomics serves two main goals: reducing the side effects of medicines, and increasing their efficacy. Therefore, overall advances in this technology are very valuable and desirable. However, as with any new technology, it raises many controversies:

(1) **Disincentives to Develop Drugs for Small Groups of Patients** — The development of new drugs costs a lot of money, and pharmaceutical companies have little incentive to develop drugs that can be sold to only a small cross-section of the population. As a result, most existing drugs will be tailored to patients with the most common genetic variations, and only a few customized drugs will be available to treat a particular disease. Therefore, some patients may be left with no suitable drug choice, should their genetic makeup render them non-responsive to an existing drug. Unarguably, this is sad. However, pharmacogenomics by itself does not make drugs unavailable to smaller groups of patients. What it does is warn in advance that particular drugs will not work for these patients or, worse, might even be toxic. This can save money and can spare these patients from unnecessary adverse drug reactions.

(2) **Individualized Rates for Health Insurance** — Pharmacogenomics requires knowledge of the genetic makeup of each individual. Some diseases are already associated with specific SNPs and genetic makeup. Even more diseases will be associated with specific SNPs in the future. Therefore, it will soon be possible to predict the susceptibility of each individual person to many diseases. For example, the deCODE Genetics company, located in Iceland, already offers a test for the genetic risks of 48 diseases and traits, ranging from heart attack and diabetes, to alcohol flush reaction and male pattern baldness, for a cost of only US$1,100. Insurance companies may use this knowledge to estimate the possible cost for the healthcare of each individual. Therefore, they could apply insurance rates based on an individual's genetic profile. Although it may sound controversial, it could be the appropriate thing to do. That said, there may be a role for legislative protection against "genetic discrimination." In the US, there is already such federal legislation in place, called GINA: the Genetic Information Nondiscrimination Act of 2008.

(3) **A Gap between Rich and Poor Countries** — Newly-developed drugs might have differing marketplace penetration in poor versus

rich countries. Pharmacogenomics would be primarily used in richer developed countries, and lead to the development of drugs tailored to specific genetic subgroups of people. In developing countries, on the other hand, there is a shortage of even generic drugs. Therefore, the priority in developing countries will still remain to create drugs for large populations, rather than development of pharmacogenomics that helps to tailor drugs for subgroups.

Future

Pharmacogenomics is already present in everyday life. For example, already in 2008, it was estimated that ~25% of all outpatients in the US received one or more drugs having pharmacogenomic information in the label for that drug.[11] The possible benefits of pharmacogenomics are obvious. However, this technology is still in its infancy. It will probably take another several years until all SNPs are mapped out and associated with drug behaviors in the body. The efficacy and the safety of several drugs can already be predicted using existing pharmacogenomical tests. The accuracy of such predictions is significant. For example, a test from deCODE Genetics that predicts whether asthma patients will respond to steroid treatment has more than 90% accuracy. As this technology develops, tests will become even more accurate and valuable, helping to bring pharmacogenomics into mainstream clinical practice.

Eventually, drugs will be prescribed based on a patient's genetic profile. At first, patients will be divided into groups based on their SNP pattern, and predictions will be possible only for large groups with similar genetic makeups. However, in the future, predictions will be possible for smaller and smaller groups, until they might become completely individualized. An estimated 2.3 million SNPs will eventually have to be analyzed to decide which drugs and what doses will work the best for each individual patient. It will not be possible to do it manually, so computer programs will have to be created to facilitate this type of analysis.

Ideally, all SNPs in the genome of each patient should be mapped, and the information made available to doctors. Then, each time a doctor has to render a decision regarding the patient's treatment, he/she will run a computer analysis to figure out which drugs and what doses will work best for each individual. This can probably be automated into electronic health record technology, so that when an electronic prescription is written, the software can automatically consult the patient's personal genetic database and inform the doctor of any potential issues. It will take, however, some time (at least 10 years) before this will be widely practiced, because the cost of analysis is currently too high. Also, doctors are not yet familiar and ready to perform such analysis. Nevertheless, the cost of DNA sequencing and SNP analysis is falling fast. Recently, next-generation DNA sequencers have been developed,[12] and it is now feasible that the DNA sequencing of a whole human genome could come down to more reasonable cost of US$1,000.[13]

Not only will pharmacogenomics help in decisions about existing drug choices, it will also help to develop new drugs. The study of genetic polymorphisms and the mapping of SNPs will help identify genes that are involved in one's susceptibility to diseases. Once a gene associated with a disease is identified, the mechanisms of its functions in the body can be studied, and its relationship to the disease can be understood. In turn, this will help identify new drugs that can target the gene. It is currently estimated that the human genome might reveal about 8,000 novel targets — quite an impressive number! For comparison, at the end of the last century, only 483 target molecules for drugs were known.

Besides variations of nucleotides in the DNA sequence, which are responsible for SNPs, gene expression can be changed by other modifications, such as methylation of DNA, and acetylation of proteins that bind to DNA. In fact, recent studies show that most of the human genome serves to regulate gene expression, while less than 2% represents the actual genes that carry instructions for making proteins.[6] The science that analyses such modifications is called epigenetics or epigenomics, while such modifications are called epigenetic modifications. Since epigenetic modifications can alter gene expression and, as a result, the levels of proteins, they also can change how drugs are processed in our bodies. Thus, epigenetic analysis can provide valuable data for pharmacogenomics. For example, it is estimated that out of around 300 genes involved in drug metabolism, almost 60 can be regulated by DNA methylation.[14] The branch of pharmacogenomics that deals with epigenetics is called pharmacoepigenomics. Although pharmacoepigenomics is still in its infancy, its further development is necessary for the complete understanding of drug behavior in the body and for future medicine.

References

1. Lazarou J, Pomeranz BH, Corey PN. (1998) Incidence of adverse drug reactions in hospitalized patients: a meta-analysis of prospective studies. *JAMA* **279:** 1200–5.
2. Motulsky AG. (1957) Drug reactions enzymes, and biochemical genetics. *JAMA* **165:** 835–7.
3. Vogel F. (1959) Moderne Probleme der Humangenetik. *Ergeb Inn Med U Kinderheilk* **12:** 52–125.
4. Thomas DL, *et al.* (2009) Genetic variation in IL28B and spontaneous clearance of hepatitis C virus. *Nature* **461:** 798–801.
5. Ge D, *et al.* (2009) Genetic variation in IL28B predicts hepatitis C treatment-induced viral clearance. *Nature* **461:** 399–401.
6. Bernstein BE, *et al.* (2012) An integrated encyclopedia of DNA elements in the human genome. *Nature* **489:** 57–74.
7. Hindorff LA, *et al.* (2009) Potential etiologic and functional implications of genome-wide association loci for human diseases and traits. *Proc Natl Acad Sci USA* **106:** 9362–7.
8. Zanger UM, Turpeinen M, Klein K, Schwab M. (2008) Functional pharmacogenetics/genomics of human cytochromes P450 involved in drug biotransformation. *Anal Bioanal Chem* **392:** 1093–108.
9. Janne PA, Johnson BE. (2006) Effect of epidermal growth factor receptor tyrosine kinase domain mutations on the outcome of patients with non-small cell lung cancer treated with epidermal growth factor receptor tyrosine kinase inhibitors. *Clin Cancer Res* **12:** 4416s–4420s.
10. Farbstein D, *et al.* (2011) Vitamin E therapy results in a reduction in HDL function in individuals with diabetes and the haptoglobin 2-1 genotype. *Atherosclerosis* **219:** 240–4.
11. Frueh, FW, *et al.* (2008) Pharmacogenomic biomarker information in drug labels approved by the United States food and drug administration: prevalence of related drug use. *Pharmacotherapy* **28:** 992–8.

12. Pushkarev D, Neff NF, Quake SR. (2009) Single-molecule sequencing of an individual human genome. *Nat Biotechnol* **27:** 847–50.
13. Trent RJ. (2010) Pathology practice and pharmacogenomics. *Pharmacogenomics* **11:** 105–11.
14. Kacevska M, Ivanov M, Ingelman-Sundberg M. (2011) Perspectives on epigenetics and its relevance to adverse drug reactions. *Clin Pharmacol Ther* **89:** 902–7.

CHAPTER 7

Other Technologies

In previous chapters, several innovative technologies that promise to advance the future of medicine have been described. Many new technologies and techniques are being developed as this book is being written (for example, epigenetic therapies). By the time this is read, medicine may already have advanced. On the other hand, the merging of already existing technologies also provides opportunities for new medical treatments. Here are some of the most promising new developments.

Robotics

Advances in robotics open up possibilities for the creation of artificial systems which could simulate human cells and organs. It is possible that in the future, damaged tissues or organs will be replaced with artificial ones. One example of this is the "closed loop" insulin delivery system, which can also be viewed as an artificial or bionic pancreas. This implantable system consists of three parts: the glucose sensor (described in Chapter 5), the minicomputer, and the insulin pump. The sensor constantly measures glucose levels in the blood and sends data to the minicomputer. Then, as insulin levels fluctuate, the computer calculates how much insulin is needed in the blood, and tells the pump how much insulin to deliver. Once all the "bugs" are worked out, this device will essentially cure type 1 diabetes. Such a device, manufactured by Medtronic Inc., is currently under review for approval in the US and already approved in 50 countries.[1] The very latest studies demonstrated that an artificial pancreas such as this provides better glycaemic control than conventional insulin pump therapy.[2,3]

Robotics can also be used to enhance our natural organs. For example, scientists recently created a costume that can help disabled and elderly people walk and lift heavy objects. This costume, called a "hybrid assistive limb" (HAL), was developed by Japanese specialists and made commercially available in 2005. The most advanced model of the costume, HAL 3, represents a metal "exoskeleton" that can be placed on the patient's feet and help with walking. The costume has an engine, controlled by two "bio-cybernetic" systems. The first system registers signals about the patient's intentions to move, which are transmitted from the brain to muscle. When a person wants to move, the brain sends an electric signal to the muscles, through the nerves that lie under the skin of the feet. Then, sensors attached to the skin register the signals and send them to a computer, which transforms the nerve signals into electrical signals that control the engine. The second "bio-cybernetic" system controls the engines that coordinate the body's movements, and is auto-activated as soon as the user begins to move.

Recent progress in vision restoration is another illustration of how robotics can be used to advance medicine. An American company called Second Sight has recently achieved very impressive results: It has developed a retinal prosthesis for the blind, which basically represents the first step toward the manufacturing of artificial eyes. Using a miniature camera that is installed in the patient's glasses, this prosthesis system captures video images and converts them into a series of small electrical pulses that are then wirelessly transmitted to an array of electrodes on the retina. The cells still remaining in damaged retinas are then stimulated by these pulses, which causes the perception of patterns of light in the brain. Eventually, patients learn to interpret these visual patterns and gain some functional vision. Thirty patients have already participated in the clinical trial. The study concluded that most subjects with profound visual loss perform better on visual tasks with the system than without it, and the long-term safety of Second Sight's retinal prosthesis system is acceptable.[4] The system's latest model is Argus II. A group of scientists from the US and France recently reported that, using this model, text can successfully be stimulated and read as visual Braille in retinal prosthesis patients.[5] This "bionic eye" is already commercially available in Europe for around $115,000, and was recently recommended for FDA approval in the US. However, this device has certain limitations: It can help only patients who had vision and then lost it due to disease or injury, but cannot help people who were born blind. In order for this "eye" to work, patients must have visual memory about objects, and their retina must retain at least some number of healthy cells.

These developments in "bionic eye" engineering will make it possible not just to restore, but even to enhance vision. For example, cameras that detect infrared light could be used instead of regular ones in order to achieve infrared (ability to see in the dark) vision.

The above described achievements in the medical application of robotics were facilitated by neuro-technological progress, which made it possible to transform electrical signals from devices into the neuronal signals of the body. In reverse, the process of transforming signals from the body into commands for devices is also possible. This even includes the possibility of controlling robotic devices using the power of thoughts. Recently, a team of neuroscientists, working closely with computer scientists and robotics experts, created mind-controlled robot arms.[6] Experimenting on two individuals with long-standing tetraplegia (a paralysis that results in the partial or total loss of use of all limbs and the torso), the team demonstrated that the patients were able to use a robotic arm to perform three-dimensional reach and grasp movements. Participants controlled the arm and hand over a broad space without explicit training, using signals decoded from a small region of the brain. One of the study participants, implanted with the sensor five years earlier, also used a robotic arm to drink coffee from a bottle. Although the robotic reach and grasp actions were neither as fast nor accurate as those of an able-bodied person, the results demonstrated the feasibility of movement restoration for people with an injured central nervous system. Such progress will further facilitate the manufacture of devices that can bypass neuro-signals (as in the case of nerve injury), making even such devastating conditions as paralysis following a spinal cord injury, brainstem stroke, amyotrophic lateral sclerosis and similar disorders, things of the past.

Another interesting application of robotics in medicine would be the creation of robot-doctors. In the US, NASA has recently designed a portable "robot surgeon." This portable machine is controlled over the internet by a human surgeon from a long distance away, and can be used in situations when human surgeons are not available. For example, it could be used to treat astronauts/cosmonauts in space, wounded soldiers on battlefields, or sick patients in remote areas of the world where surgeons are scarce.

Preimplantation Genetic Diagnosis

Preimplantation Genetic Diagnosis (PGD) is a technology whose progress is facilitated by advances in two main fields: *in vitro* fertilization technology, and molecular genetics. The PGD test identifies genetic defects in embryos before implanting them into the uterus, and is used in combination with *in vitro* fertilization. If a genetic defect is found in the *in vitro* created embryo, such an embryo would not be used. PGD testing is recommended when certain genetic defects in the embryo are suspected, such as those expected from couples in which at least one partner has a family history of genetic disease, in women 35 years and older, and also in couples with repeated *in vitro* fertilization failures.

PGD was first used in the UK in the 1980s, and is now being performed in many countries. By the year 2004, PGD was performed on about 7,000 embryos and resulted into more than 1,000 infants being born all around the world.[7] It became possible due to new advances in molecular genetics and reproductive technology. Molecular genetics has made it possible to link certain gene mutations to diseases, while reproductive technology has made *in vitro* fertilization possible. As *in vitro* fertilization becomes readily available and popular, more centers will perform PGD on embryos, to make sure that they are unaffected by genetic defects, and that only healthy embryos are selected for implantation.

PGD testing is usually performed on embryos consisting of six to eight cells. One or two cells from such an embryo are taken for analysis, while the remaining cells in the embryo can still divide and form a normal baby. A cell taken from the embryo is analyzed for either gene mutations or for chromosomal aberrations, depending on which familiar genetic disease is expected. If a sex-linked disorder is expected, the cell is analyzed to establish the sex of the embryo. Then, only an embryo unaffected by the expected genetic disease is selected for implantation for pregnancy. As a result, PDG ensures that newborn babies will have no familiar genetic diseases, and helps reduce the frequency of such diseases being passed on to the next generations. A number of diseases are caused by genetic defects. For example, cancers are associated with mutations of more than 30 known genes.[8] As scientists find more genetic defects that cause diseases, PGD will become even more useful.

Computational Biology (Bioinformatics)

Knowledge of biology and medicine is growing exponentially. Currently, about half a million articles are published in medicine-related fields every year. No single human brain could possibly absorb all this information. Information accumulation is growing especially fast in the field of biology that studies genes (genomics). This has been facilitated by new techniques, such as gene microarray assays (or gene chip technology). To digest all this data and to make sense of it, computer analysis will become more and more necessary in the future. As new techniques and data are accumulated in research, certain advances will reach medical practice. As a result, medical practice will become more complex and also require computer analysis. The most immediate need for computer analysis in medicine will probably be in the field of pharmacogenomics (see Chapter 6), when large numbers of SNPs must be analyzed before doctors can prescribe appropriate pharmacologic treatments.

A recent article in *The New York Times* raises the possibility that computers may not just help doctors, but rather replace them.[9] As the article points out, software programs have been assisting medical professionals since the 1970s. These programs constantly improve, becoming more and more valuable. In addition, while medical knowledge accumulates exponentially, most physicians have very little time to read medical literature after they finish their education. Computer programs, on the other hand, can analyze thousands of textbook and scientific articles every second.

Although it is not perfected yet, one such program, I.B.M.'s Watson for Healthcare, can already understand the nature of a question, read a patient's electronic record, review literature, and finally, suggest an appropriate treatment. In 1996, the Deep Blue chess program from I.B.M. claimed victory over the world's best player of the time. Why can't a program outthink a doctor in the future?

Computer technology can also open up unprecedented opportunities in the science of the brain. This, however, will not be simple. Nobody has yet a complete understanding of how the brain works. The brain is not just a rigid information storage device. It is a highly adjustable organ that processes and analyzes information. This plasticity is provided not just by a large number of neurons in the brain, but also by numerous intra-neuronal connections (synapses), which form and disintegrate constantly. It is estimated that the human brain contains about 100 billion neurons that form about 100 trillion synapses. The current believe is that these 100 trillion appearing and disappearing synapses form memory, behavior, consciousness and something that is called human mind. Modern computers are still far from reaching the power of the brain for the next two reasons.

First, they use too much energy as compared to the brain. In fact, even the brain itself is considered to be a too much energy-consuming structure; for example, for the same mass, it requires about ten times more energy than muscles. This is one of the reasons of why most animals have a very small brain — they simply cannot afford it energetically. Modern computers are much less efficient than the brain. While consuming a lot of energy, they produce a lot of heat, and heat dissipation is an important limiting factor of modern computer chips. Second, modern computers have no plasticity, and their behavior is pretty much molded into them. Both these obstacles, however, may soon be overcome. In 2014, IBM reported a new chip that functions more like a brain.[10]

This chip, named TrueNorth, contains 5.4 billion transistors and consumes only 70 milliwatts of energy. For comparison, a standard chip in modern computers contains about 1.4 billion transistors that consume up to 140 watts, which is 2000 times more. Interestingly, the new chip makes only about one thousand mathematical operations per second, as compared to billions operations per second in standard microprocessors. However, because the new chip has a large number of circuits working in parallel, it can perform 46 billion operations a second per one watt of consumed energy. These new chips can signal one to another when some type of data is registered; for example, light. Then, working in parallel, they can analyze the data and organize them into certain patterns; for example, color and shape of the light. Thus, they can recognize and interpret videos, sounds, etc. similarly to the brain. Nonetheless, this new chip is still far from human brain power. It is only the first step in the right direction, and many technological companies are working in this direction already. Giants like Microsoft, Apple and Google are working hard to develop pattern-recognizing computers that would improve their speech and photo services. In fact, computer speech recognition is already approaching human abilities. It is estimated, however, that such speech recognition requires only about 0.01% of the human brain capability, suggesting that modern computers must be about 10,000 times more powerful to fully achieve human brain capabilities.

Many academic and private institutions around the world are working to create more powerful and efficient computer chips. For example, researchers at RMIT University in Australia have developed a data storage nanostructure the memory of which depends on its past experiences. The new chip is created using a film that is more than 10,000 thinner than a human hair. The European Union assigned as much as €1 billion for the Human Brain Project aiming to reconstruct the brain in a supercomputer and eventually produce a synthetic mind. But even bigger resources are now pouring into this field of science. As mentioned above, big technological companies are currently working to imitate the functions of the brain. The military also joined the quest. For example, the described above TrueNorth computer chip was developed for drone technology using money from Pentagon. Taken together, the military and technological giants control most of the world financial resources. With all the resources directed to this field, there is a good chance that the last frontier of the human body, the brain, will soon be understood and its functions will be artificially simulated.

Some specialists forecast that by the year 2020, there will be machines that possess emotions and even consciousness. Others predict that by the year 2050, supercomputers capable of storing the entire information content of the human brain will be constructed. Regardless of how exact these estimations are, it is widely agreed that such computers can be created in the not-too-distant future.

If this comes true, it would open up new possibilities for the repair and enhancement of the human brain. Also, if the entire content of the brain could be transferred into a computer, the conscience would live longer than the body, maybe even being stored or transferred forever. Then the question would be raised: Is this a way for humans to become immortal? What is human death? Also, should one even care to treat or cure diseases? Would it not be simpler just to transfer the brain content into a new body or machine? This further raises questions about the very nature of future medicine, and may completely change medical practices as they are known today. Now, as a reminder: All futurologists agree that computers capable of storing the entire information content of the human brain will be constructed no later than the year 2050. Although, it has to be noted, even if this is at all possible, decoding the information stored in the human brain may be a big challenge.

Imagine this: In the year 2066, there is a young man named Peter. At age 36, he was hit by motorbike. His body is crippled, his spine broken and liver failing. Peter does not want to die yet, nor does he want to go through painful medical procedures. When his aunt was struck by cancer two years ago, she requested her body be cremated, and her brain information stored in banks at local hospitals. She asked Peter to authorize the transfer of her brain info into a robotic copy of her body as soon as the cost of such copy production dropped to affordable levels. Peter's aunt was not rich, and the cost is still way too high for her, even more so for Peter. Peter stared into the rainy sky through the hospital window, weighing his options…

Most people have some kind of religious beliefs, and most religions recognize the existence of the soul. Thus, most people believe that each human has a soul. However, what the soul is, and whether it resides in the brain — no one knows. Therefore, the transfer of a person's brain information into a computer may not be sufficient to transfer the whole person, and whether the transfer of a person from a body to a device will be possible remains a big question.

References

1. Bardin J. (2012) Trial of artificial pancreas gives diabetes patients a break. *Los Angeles Times,* June 12, 2012.
2. Russell SJ, *et al.* (2014) Outpatient glycemic control with a bionic pancreas in type 1 diabetes. *N Engl J Med* **371:** 313–25.
3. Haidar A, *et al.* (2014) Comparison of dual-hormone artificial pancreas, single-hormone artificial pancreas, and conventional insulin pump therapy for glycaemic control in patients with type 1 diabetes: an open-label randomised controlled crossover trial. *Lancet Diabetes Endocrinol* **3:** 17–26.
4. Humayun MS, *et al.* (2012) Interim results from the international trial of Second Sight's visual prosthesis. *Ophthalmology* **119:** 779–88.
5. Lauritzen TZ, *et al.* (2012) Reading visual braille with a retinal prosthesis. *Front Neurosci* **6:** 168.
6. Hochberg LR, *et al.* (2012) Reach and grasp by people with tetraplegia using a neurally controlled robotic arm. *Nature* **485:** 372–5.
7. Verlinsky Y, *et al.* (2004) Over a decade of experience with preimplantation genetic diagnosis: a multicenter report. *Fertil Steril* **82:** 292–4.
8. Garber JE, Offit K. (2005) Hereditary cancer predisposition syndromes. *J Clin Oncol* **23:** 276–92.
9. Hafner K. (2012) Could a Computer Outthink This Doctor? *The New York Times,* Dec 4, 2012.
10. Merolla PA, Arthur JV, Alvarez-Icaza R, *et al.* (2014) Artificial brains. A million spiking-neuron integrated circuit with a scalable communication network and interface. *Science* **345:** 668–73.

CHAPTER 8

Modern Science and Dietary Supplements

Whether or not they should, dietary supplements play an important role in modern life. For example, more than half of adult Americans take supplements in the hope of improving their health, spending about $27 billion per year. Chinese consumers spend even more, with amounts projected to reach 600 billion yuan (about $100 billion) by 2015. Therefore, this book would not be complete without considering their effects on health. People take supplements for many reasons: to lose weight, to improve physical appearance or athletic performance, to avoid using prescription drugs, to slow down aging, and to stay healthier overall. New supplements that promise miracles enter the market every year. However, recent studies point out that they have very little value to health, if any. In many cases, they have shockingly dangerous side effects.

Definition

A dietary supplement is a preparation containing nutrients (such as vitamins, minerals, amino acids, extracts, etc.), intended to maintain or improve health. According to the Codex Alimentarius Commission (sponsored by the World Health Organization), dietary supplements are food. Although many countries define them as food, others classify them as drugs; thus, the definition of a dietary supplement varies depending on country. In the US, according to the Dietary Supplement Health and Education Act of 1994, it is a product containing any of the following: vitamins, minerals, herbs/botanicals (excluding tobacco), amino acids, any substance histori-cally used to supplement the diet, or formulations of any of the above. In addition, it must meet the following criteria: (a) intended for ingestion in pill, powder or liquid form; (b) not represented for use as a conventional food; (c) labeled "dietary supplement."

Regulations

Most countries place dietary supplements in the category of food rather than drugs, which means that manufacturers, not the government, are responsible for ensuring their safety. However, since the latest studies reveal potentially harmful effects of supplements, governments around the world are stepping up regulations to minimize such effects. The European Union considers supplements food, but its Directive 2002/46/EC from 2002 requires that they demonstrate safety in purity and dosage. Nonetheless, some Europeans, especially in the UK, disagree with such requirements, arguing that they restrict consumer choice and freedom. The situation is different in the US, where governmental agencies (such as the FDA) must demonstrate that a supplement is unsafe in order to prohibit its sale, versus requiring proof of supplement safety from the manufacturer. At the same time, governmental agencies are not sufficiently funded to do this job, which leaves American consumers less protected against the potentially dangerous effects of supplements. In fact, it is estimated that the FDA has identified only 1–10% of all adverse effects caused by supplements.[1]

In both the US and the EU, supplements cannot claim to cure or treat a disease. If they do, they are considered drugs and require appropriate government approvals. However, this is very difficult to regulate, especially on commercial internet websites. For example, the dietary supplement hydrazine sulfate, sold in the US, claims to treat cancer, despite the absence of evidence for its effectiveness or safety.[2] Regulation is even more difficult for supplements sold from consumer-to-consumer or by word of mouth, as practiced by companies such as Herbalife. Even worse, according to Consumer Reports,[3] until 2007, supplement makers in the US did not have to inform the FDA if they received reports of serious adverse effects, an obligation long-required for prescription drugs. After the appropriate laws took effect, the FDA received 1,359 reports of serious adverse effects from manufacturers, and 602 from consumers in just the two following years. This publication also cited the Natural Medicines Comprehensive Database, which shows that only about a third of supplement products have some level of effectiveness supported by science, and that close to 12% of them have been linked to either safety or quality concerns.

Health Effects

The idea behind taking supplements is very simple. When people learned that vitamins and minerals are essential to the body, and that their shortage can cause dysfunctions and diseases, people began taking them to avoid such dysfunctions and diseases. When people discovered that diseases and aging are associated with increased oxidation in the body, they began taking antioxidants, with the hope of preventing or stopping diseases and aging. This could work and be just fine if one knew exactly how much of a supplement is missing in the body, which itself depends upon the genetic makeup and food intake of each individual. However, since they can do such great things for the body, people just decided that more supplements = better! As strange as it sounds, not many questioned if more could be too much, or if too much could be unhealthy. Now, new studies reveal that taking supplements, even the most common ones, can ruin our health. Below are few examples.

(1) **Vitamins** — In general, a vitamin is defined as an organic compound that is required by, but cannot be synthesized by, an organism in sufficient quantities. Thus, vitamins must be obtained from food. They facilitate chemical reactions, and the body requires that certain vitamins are present at certain times. If there is a serious deficiency in one or more of these compounds, a disease or even a permanent damage can occur. Vitamins are classified as either water-soluble or fat-soluble. Humans require 13 of them: nine water-soluble (eight B vitamins and one C vitamin) and four fat-soluble (A, D, E, and K). However, in large doses, vitamins have been documented to have side-effects such as nausea, diarrhea, and vomiting. Because the body can get rid of an excess of water-soluble vitamins (with urine) easier than fat-soluble vitamins, the chance of poisoning by fat-soluble

vitamins is higher than that by water-soluble ones. However, besides those immediate side-effects, vitamin overloads can also have long-term damaging effects on health.

The general belief used to be that an increased intake of vitamins would improve overall health, which might also lead to longer lives. But studies published so far demonstrate that this assumption is false. In the best case, multivitamin use has been found to have no effect on mortality,[4,5] while other studies have shown that vitamin A and E supplementation not only provides no benefits for healthy individuals, but may actually increase mortality,[6] especially in those individuals who smoke.

Another hope was that vitamins, especially those that possess antioxidant properties (such as vitamin A, C and E), can help fight disease. However, studies demonstrate that this is also not the case. For example, a study of 160,000 post-menopausal women found that multivitamin supplementation prevented neither cancer, heart attack, nor stroke.[4] Another, even larger study, involving more than 180,000 participants, also found no association between multivitamin use and reduced cardiovascular disease, cancer, or overall morbidity.[5] Also, multivitamin use is not associated with a significantly increased or decreased risk of breast cancer.[7] There is a widespread belief that vitamin C mega doses can help fight cold infections; however, a 2001 study from the Australian National University demonstrated that they neither reduce a cold's duration, nor its severity.[8] In evidence contrary to what was expected, vitamin supplementation may have harmful effects. A study published in 2009 found that vitamins C and E may curb some benefits of exercise.[9] A double-blind trial published in 2011 found that vitamin E increases the risk of prostate cancer in healthy men.[10]

(2) **Aspirin** — Although aspirin is a drug, many people take it daily as a supplement, without apparent medical reason, but just to keep in good health; thus, its use as a supplement will be considered here. Aspirin is one of the most widely used drugs in the world and is used to treat a number of conditions, such as pain, headache, fever, heart attacks, strokes, and others. However, very often, doctors recommend that their patients take a daily "baby dose" (81 mg) of aspirin to keep in better health. Indeed, aspirin is probably the most versatile and multifunctional compound, and

has been shown to improve a number of conditions. At least three publications in 2012 have reported that its regular supplementation can even prevent cancers and the risk of metastasis.[11–13] Nevertheless, as miraculous as aspirin is, its daily supplementation still can cause some dangerous side effects. First, since aspirin is an acid (acetylsalicylic acid), it has a negative effect on the stomach lining, and thus is not recommended for individuals with ulcers or gastritis. Second, some individuals are allergic to it. Third, it can be harmful for people with certain conditions. For example, it inhibits the kidneys' ability to excrete uric acid, and can harm people with kidney disease, gout, and hyperuricemia. It can cause anemia in individuals with the genetic disease called glucose-6-phosphate dehydrogenase deficiency. Also, aspirin should not be given to children and adolescents during episodes of fever, as this has been linked with Reye's syndrome. Thus, aspirin supplementation requires many precautions.

(3) **Calcium** — Calcium is essential for the body. It gets replenished through food. The main portion of calcium is used by the body for the mineralization of bones and teeth. Long-term deficiency of calcium can lead to a softening of bones in children, and poor blood clotting in adults. In the elderly, and especially in menopausal women, it can lead to osteoporosis — the condition of bone deterioration that leads to an increased risk of fractures. Therefore, doctors routinely recommend that older people take calcium supplements.

Although approximately 99% of the body's calcium is stored in the bones and teeth, a very important fact is currently overlooked: It is found in every cell of the body, where it plays a crucial role in the regulation of a number of molecules (for example, phosphotases and kinases) and cell functions.[14] Thus, it is not surprising that calcium excess can disrupt normal physiological pathways and cause harm. For example, high calcium intake was related to advanced prostate cancer.[15] It can cause belching, stomach gas, and decrease the effectiveness of several drugs. It was also related to the development of kidney stones, but this was later disproved by more research. Also, it has been recently found that calcium supplementation puts people at a greater risk for heart attacks.[16] This may be due to the fact that swallowing a calcium pill once a day can lead to a sudden increase in calcium levels in the body, as opposed to getting calcium through regular food, which is normally taken a few times a day and releases calcium into the body more slowly. Regardless of the reasons for these dangerous side effects, it is clear that calcium can harm, and there is a need to rethink the approach regarding calcium supplementation.

(4) **Other Supplements** — Consumer Reports states that of more than 54,000 dietary supplements in the Natural Medicines Comprehensive Database, only about a third have some level of safety and effectiveness supported by scientific evidence, and close to 12% have been linked to safety concerns or problems with product quality.[3] A number of commonly taken supplements can have serious side effects (please see Tables 8.1 and 8.2). In addition, most supplements can reduce the effectiveness of certain medications. For example, calcium can decrease the effectiveness of certain antibiotics and other drugs.[17] Vitamin D might reduce the effectiveness of atorvastatin (lipitor), other heart medications, birth-control pills, and HIV/AIDS drugs.[3] And as we learn more, more dangerous side effects of dietary supplements are discovered. What science is saying is that any supplement may have harmful side effects, and extreme caution should be used before taking any of them.

Why Dietary Supplements Harm

As shown, virtually all supplements hide some risks to health. There may be several reasons why they can harm:

(1) **Overly High Doses** — Many pills contain either 100% of the daily dose of one or several supplements, or even higher doses. Unless we are starving or are living in poor conditions with very limited choices of food, normal foods already contain 100% of all nutrients needed. Taking extra supplements leads to an excess of normal doses.

(2) **Absorption in a Short Time** — When getting nutrients through food, they are taken a few times a day, which would be equivalent to taking supplements a few times a day. In addition, as food is digested and absorbed more slowly than just a small pill, nutrients from food enter the blood stream slower than from a single pill. Thus, a once-a-day intake of

supplements can cause a sudden spike, followed by a sudden drop of their levels in the body.

(3) **Quality and Contaminations** — Most supplements are either extracted or synthesized in factories, which involves chemical treatments and purifications. If contaminated and not sufficiently purified, supplements may contain some chemicals that are dangerous for health. This processing requires that manufacturers implement good manufacturing practices (GMP), which is not the case. In fact, it is estimated that about 70% of supplement manufacturers do not comply with GMP. Governmental agencies around the world try to enforce GMP; but, in most countries, they are grossly underfunded to do this job. Thus, it is better to buy supplements from trusted sources. Also, the quality of many supplements can be verified on the website of the non-profit organization US Pharmacopeia (USP).

(4) **Enhancing Both Positive and Negative Things at the Same Time** — (a) if supplements improve the functions of normal cells, they can also improve the functions of cancerous cells, thus promoting cancer growth; (b) supplements such as antioxidants can often be a double-edged sword in the body. Since they reduce the number of free radicals, which normally can damage cells, they also reduce the effectiveness of some anticancer chemotherapies; (c) not all free radicals are bad for the body — some of them serve in cell signaling and normal functioning; thus, eliminating free radicals completely may dis-regulate cell functions; (d) human cells produce a number of antioxidants and, if we take overly high doses of antioxidants via supplementation, the body may sense this and shut down its natural defenses as unnecessary things; (e) some dietary supplements exhibit both antioxidant and pro-oxidant properties simultaneously; for example, vitamin C.[54]

Conclusion

An avalanche of information regarding dietary supplements is published every year, and understanding their effects on health can be complicated. For example, the results of more than 100 studies on the health effects of

Table 8.1   Common Dietary Supplements

Name	Recommended Uses	Reported Efficiencies	Contraindications	Concerns and Dangers
Vitamin E	General health	May be of benefit against age-related macular degeneration,[18] but not against cancer or major cardiovascular diseases.[19] Reports of its use against neurological diseases are inconsistent.	Smokers	Associated with increased risk of heart failure,[19] and may increase bleeding, diarrhea and nausea. Can exacerbate upper respiratory infections.[22]
Chondroitin	Osteoarthritis	Helps in osteoarthritis treatment.[20,21]	Should not be taken by children and pregnant or nursing women.	May enhance effects of anticoagulant drugs.[23] May cause mild diarrhea and nausea.
Glucosamine	Osteoarthritis	Helps in hip[20] and knee[21] osteoarthritis treatment.	Should not be taken by diabetic people and by pregnant or nursing women.	May cause heartburn and diarrhea.
Human growth hormone	Enhancement of performance and appearance	There is no scientific evidence of the claims.	Should not be taken by children, pregnant or nursing women, diabetic people, and people with cancer.	Linked to colorectal cancer[24] and leukemia.[25] May cause dyspepsia, diarrhea and nausea.

(*Continued*)

Table 8.1   (*Continued*)

Name	Recommended Uses	Reported Efficiencies	Contraindications	Concerns and Dangers
L-glutamine	Implement of concentration, alertness and memory.	There is no scientific evidence of the claims.	Should not be taken by pregnant or nursing women and people with renal or hepatic failure.	May contribute to chronic neurodegeneration in several disorders and to the brain damage occurring acutely after status epilepticus, cerebral ischemia or traumatic brain injury.[26,27]

Table 8.2   Common Herbal Dietary Supplements

Name	Recommended Uses	Reported Efficiencies	Contraindications	Concerns and Dangers
Ephedra (*Ephedra sinica*)	Weight loss	Promotes weight loss.[28,29]	Pregnancy, psychiatric disorders, glaucoma, cardiovascular disease, hypertension, diabetes, thyroid disorders, and others.	Sudden death,[38–40] stroke,[39,41,42] myocardial infarction,[39,42] dizziness,[42] psychosis,[43,44] mania[45] and others.
Ginkgo (*Ginkgo biloba*)	Memory enhancement	May be neuroprotective in ischemia stroke[30] and effective in the treatment of dementia associated with Alzheimer's disease.[31,32]	Should not be taken by children, pregnant or nursing women, diabetic people, and people with hematological disorders, epilepsy and seizures.	No credible reports of danger, but may be contaminated with colchicines,[46] which are harmful for human health. May interact with anticoagulant drugs.[47]

(*Continued*)

Table 8.2 (*Continued*)

Name	Recommended Uses	Reported Efficiencies	Contraindications	Concerns and Dangers
St. John's wort (*Hypericum perforatum*)	Depression	May be effective for the treatment of mild to moderate depression,[33] but not major depression.[34]	Pregnancy, nursing, pending surgery.	Interferes with most drugs,[48] including indinavir,[49] irinotecan,[50] warfarin, phenprocoumon, cyclosporin, HIV protease inhibitors, theophylline, digoxin and oral contraceptives.[51] Endangers the success of organ transplantation.[52]
Valerian (*Valeriana officinalis*)	Anxiety, insomnia	The evidence is inconclusive for both anxiety and insomnia.[35-37]	Pregnancy, nursing, pending surgery.	May damage liver.[53]

plants from the Ginseng group, which includes about 20 species (Chinese ginseng, Korean ginseng, Siberian ginseng, etc.) have been published in 2012 alone. In these publications, Ginseng is suggested to inhibit cancers,[55–59] prevent heart failure,[60–62] control blood sugar levels[63–65] and blood pressure,[66] protect against influenza viral infections,[67,68] inhibit inflammation,[69,70] be neuroprotective,[71] improve neurocognitive functions,[72] inhibit atopic dermatitis,[73] suppress asthma[74] and suppress obesity.[75] On the other hand, also in 2012, another analysis came to the following conclusion: With the exceptions of Vitamin D and omega-3 fatty acids, there is no data to support the widespread use of dietary supplements in westernized populations; indeed, many of these supplements may be harmful.[76] All of this information is confusing, even for specialists. So, what should be made of all of this data?

It seems that most problems associated with supplements can be avoided if we simply maintain a balanced diet and just get the nutrients from regular foods. Current science and common sense suggest that supplements should be taken only when there is a true deficiency, and the benefits clearly outweigh the possible risks of supplementation. Probably, only certain groups of people should consider taking dietary supplements: (a) people with certain medical conditions (some genetic diseases, lactose intolerance and other deficiency disorders); (b) people who either diet or avoid certain food groups (vegetarians, vegans, or people who often eat processed food); (c) pregnant or lactating women; and (d) seniors. Thus, before taking any dietary supplements, one should ask if one belongs to any such group.

In traditional Chinese and some other such medicines, many natural products, including herbs, are used to treat numerous health problems and thus, could be classified as drugs. However, it seems that modern western medicine does not take these products seriously and has labeled them "dietary supplements." Some of those "supplements" may act as potent drugs. Not surprisingly, as any drug, they may interact with other drugs and produce side effects. Thus, it is warranted that some "dietary supplements" should be re-evaluated and labeled "drugs." This would help avoid the dangerous effects of dietary supplements, and improve future medicine.

References

1. Heinrich J. (2000) Adverse drug events substantial problem but magnitude uncertain: Testimony before the Committee on Health, Education, Labor, and Pensions, US Senate.
2. Black M, Hussain H. (2000) Hydrazine, cancer, the Internet, isoniazid, and the liver. *Ann Intern Med* **133:** 911–3.
3. Dangerous supplements: what you don't know about these 12 ingredients could hurt you. *Consum Rep* **75:** 16–20 (2010).
4. Neuhouser ML, *et al.* (2009) Multivitamin use and risk of cancer and cardiovascular disease in the Women's Health Initiative cohorts. *Arch Intern Med* **169:** 294–304.
5. Park SY, Murphy SP, Wilkens LR, *et al.* (2011) Multivitamin use and the risk of mortality and cancer incidence: the multiethnic cohort study. *Am J Epidemiol* **173:** 906–14.
6. Bjelakovic G, Nikolova D, Gluud LL, *et al.* (2007) Mortality in randomized trials of antioxidant supplements for primary and secondary prevention: systematic review and meta-analysis. *Jama* **297:** 842–57.
7. Chan AL, Leung HW, Wang SF. (2011) Multivitamin supplement use and risk of breast cancer: a meta-analysis. *Ann Pharmacother* **45:** 476–84.
8. Audera C, Patulny RV, Sander BH, Douglas RM. (2001) Mega-dose vitamin C in treatment of the common cold: a randomised controlled trial. *Med J Aust* **175:** 359–62.
9. Wade N. (2009) Vitamins Found to Curb Exercise Benefits. *The New York Times,* May 11, 2009.
10. Klein EA, *et al.* (2011) Vitamin E and the risk of prostate cancer: the Selenium and Vitamin E Cancer Prevention Trial (SELECT). *Jama* **306:** 1549–56.
11. Rothwell PM, *et al.* (2012) Short-term effects of daily aspirin on cancer incidence, mortality, and non-vascular death: analysis of the time course of risks and benefits in 51 randomised controlled trials. *Lancet* **379:** 1602–12.
12. Rothwell PM, *et al.* (2012) Effect of daily aspirin on risk of cancer metastasis: a study of incident cancers during randomised controlled trials. *Lancet* **379:** 1591–601.
13. Algra AM, Rothwell PM. (2012) Effects of regular aspirin on long-term cancer incidence and metastasis: a systematic comparison of evidence from observational studies versus randomised trials. *Lancet Oncol* **13:** 518–27.

14. Ermak G, Davies KJ. (2002) Calcium and oxidative stress: from cell signaling to cell death. *Mol Immunol* **38:** 713–21.

15. Giovannucci E, *et al.* (1998) Calcium and fructose intake in relation to risk of prostate cancer. *Cancer Res* **58:** 442–7.

16. Grandi NC, *et al.* (2012) Calcium, phosphate and the risk of cardiovascular events and all-cause mortality in a population with stable coronary heart disease. *Heart* **98:** 926–33.

17. Murray JJ, Healy MD. (1991) Drug-mineral interactions: a new responsibility for the hospital dietitian. *J Am Diet Assoc* **91:** 66–70, 73.

18. A randomized, placebo-controlled, clinical trial of high-dose supplementation with vitamins C and E, beta carotene, and zinc for age-related macular degeneration and vision loss: AREDS report no. 8. *Arch Ophthalmol* **119:** 1417–36 (2001).

19. Lonn E, *et al.* (2005) Effects of long-term vitamin E supplementation on cardiovascular events and cancer: a randomized controlled trial. *Jama* **293:** 1338–47.

20. McAlindon TE, LaValley MP, Gulin JP, Felson DT. (2000) Glucosamine and chondroitin for treatment of osteoarthritis: a systematic quality assessment and meta-analysis. *Jama* **283:** 1469–75.

21. Richy F, *et al.* (2003) Structural and symptomatic efficacy of glucosamine and chondroitin in knee osteoarthritis: a comprehensive meta-analysis. *Arch Intern Med* **163:** 1514–22.

22. Graat JM, Schouten EG, Kok FJ. (2002) Effect of daily vitamin E and multivitamin-mineral supplementation on acute respiratory tract infections in elderly persons: a randomized controlled trial. *Jama* **288:** 715–21.

23. Rozenfeld V, Crain JL, Callahan AK. (2004) Possible augmentation of warfarin effect by glucosamine-chondroitin. *Am J Health Syst Pharm* **61:** 306–7.

24. Swerdlow AJ, Higgins CD, Adlard P, Preece MA. (2002) Risk of cancer in patients treated with human pituitary growth hormone in the UK, 1959–85: a cohort study. *Lancet* **360:** 273–7.

25. Fradkin JE, *et al.* (1993) Risk of leukemia after treatment with pituitary growth hormone. *Jama* **270:** 2829–32.

26. Meldrum BS. (2000) Glutamate as a neurotransmitter in the brain: review of physiology and pathology. *J Nutr* **130:** 1007S–1015S.

27. Garlick PJ. (2001) Assessment of the safety of glutamine and other amino acids. *J Nutr* **131:** 2556S–2561S.

28. Boozer CN, *et al.* (2001) An herbal supplement containing Ma Huang-Guarana for weight loss: a randomized, double-blind trial. *Int J Obes Relat Metab Disord* **25:** 316–24.

29. Song MK, Um JY, Jang HJ, Lee BC. (2012) Beneficial effect of dietary Ephedra sinica on obesity and glucose intolerance in high-fat diet-fed mice. *Exp Ther Med* **3:** 707–12.

30. Zhang Z, Peng D, Zhu H, Wang X. (2012) Experimental evidence of Ginkgo biloba extract EGB as a neuroprotective agent in ischemia stroke rats. *Brain Res Bull* **87:** 193–8.

31. Wettstein A. (2000) Cholinesterase inhibitors and Gingko extracts — are they comparable in the treatment of dementia? Comparison of published placebo-controlled efficacy studies of at least six months' duration. *Phytomedicine* **6:** 393–401.

32. Oken BS, Storzbach DM, Kaye JA. (1998) The efficacy of Ginkgo biloba on cognitive function in Alzheimer disease. *Arch Neurol* **55:** 1409–15.

33. Gaster B, Holroyd J. (2000) St John's wort for depression: a systematic review. *Arch Intern Med* **160:** 152–6.

34. Effect of Hypericum perforatum (St John's wort) in major depressive disorder: a randomized controlled trial. *Jama* **287:** 1807–14 (2002).

35. Jacobs BP, Bent S, Tice JA, *et al.* (2005) An internet-based randomized, placebo-controlled trial of kava and valerian for anxiety and insomnia. *Medicine (Baltimore)* **84:** 197–207.

36. Ernst E. (2006) Herbal remedies for anxiety — a systematic review of controlled clinical trials. *Phytomedicine* **13:** 205–8.

37. Stevinson C, Ernst E. (2000) Valerian for insomnia: a systematic review of randomized clinical trials. *Sleep Med* **1:** 91–99.

38. Theoharides TC. (1997) Sudden death of a healthy college student related to ephedrine toxicity from a Ma Huang-containing drink. *J Clin Psychopharmacol* **17:** 437–9.

39. Samenuk D, *et al.* (2002) Adverse cardiovascular events temporally associated with Ma Huang, an herbal source of ephedrine. *Mayo Clin Proc* **77:** 12–6.

40. Gurley BJ, Gardner SF, White LM, Wang PL. (1998) Ephedrine pharmacokinetics after the ingestion of nutritional supplements containing Ephedra sinica (Ma Huang). *Ther Drug Monit* **20:** 439–45.

41. Bernstein E, Diskant BM. (1982) Phenylpropanolamine: a potentially hazardous drug. *Ann Emerg Med* **11:** 311–5.

42. Adverse events associated with ephedrine-containing products — Texas, December 1993–September 1995. *MMWR Morb Mortal Wkly Rep* **45:** 689–93 (1996).

43. Whitehouse AM, Duncan JM. (1987) Ephedrine psychosis rediscovered. *Br J Psychiatry* **150:** 258–61.

44. Doyle H, Kargin M. (1996) Herbal stimulant containing ephedrine has also caused psychosis. *BMJ* **313:** 756.
45. Capwell RR. (1995) Ephedrine-induced mania from an herbal diet supplement. *Am J Psychiatry* **152:** 647.
46. Petty HR, *et al.* (2001) Identification of colchicine in placental blood from patients using herbal medicines. *Chem Res Toxicol* **14:** 1254–8.
47. Taki Y, *et al.* (2012) Ginkgo biloba extract attenuates warfarin-mediated anticoagulation through induction of hepatic cytochrome P450 enzymes by bilobalide in mice. *Phytomedicine* **19:** 177–82.
48. Moore LB, *et al.* (2000) St. John's wort induces hepatic drug metabolism through activation of the pregnane X receptor. *Proc Natl Acad Sci USA* **97:** 7500–2.
49. Piscitelli SC, Burstein AH, Chaitt D, *et al.* (2000) Indinavir concentrations and St John's wort. *Lancet* **355:** 547–8.
50. Mathijssen RH, Verweij J, de Bruijn P, *et al.* (2002) Effects of St. John's wort on irinotecan metabolism. *J Natl Cancer Inst* **94:** 1247–9.
51. Henderson L, Yue QY, Bergquist C, *et al.* (2002) St John's wort (Hypericum perforatum): drug interactions and clinical outcomes. *Br J Clin Pharmacol* **54:** 349–56.
52. Ernst E. (2002) St John's Wort supplements endanger the success of organ transplantation. *Arch Surg* **137:** 316–9.
53. MacGregor FB, Abernethy VE, Dahabra S, *et al.* (1989) Hepatotoxicity of herbal remedies. *BMJ* **299:** 1156–7.
54. Podmore ID, *et al.* (1998) Vitamin C exhibits pro-oxidant properties. *Nature* **392:** 559.
55. Ji Y, *et al.* (2012) Ginsenosides extracted from nanoscale Chinese white ginseng enhances anticancer effect. *J Nanosci Nanotechnol* **12:** 6163–7.
56. Ma HY, Gao HY, Huang J, *et al.* (2012) Three new triterpenoids from Panax ginseng exhibit cytotoxicity against human A549 and Hep-3B cell lines. *J Nat Med* **66:** 576–82.
57. Du GJ, *et al.* (2012) Caspase-mediated pro-apoptotic interaction of panaxadiol and irinotecan in human colorectal cancer cells. *J Pharm Pharmacol* **64:** 727–34.
58. Hwang JW, *et al.* (2012) Mountain ginseng extract exhibits anti-lung cancer activity by inhibiting the nuclear translocation of NF-kappaB. *Am J Chin Med* **40:** 187–202.

59. Poudyal D, *et al.* (2012) A hexane fraction of American ginseng suppresses mouse colitis and associated colon cancer: anti-inflammatory and proapoptotic mechanisms. *Cancer Prev Res (Phila)* **5**: 685–96.
60. Moey M, *et al.* (2012) Ginseng reverses established cardiomyocyte hypertrophy and postmyocardial infarction-induced hypertrophy and heart failure. *Circ Heart Fail* **5**: 504–14.
61. Li HX, *et al.* (2012) The saponin of red ginseng protects the cardiac myocytes against ischemic injury *in vitro* and *in vivo*. *Phytomedicine* **19**: 477–83.
62. Kim SY, *et al.* (2012) Effects of red ginseng supplementation on menopausal symptoms and cardiovascular risk factors in postmenopausal women: a double-blind randomized controlled trial. *Menopause* **19**: 461–6.
63. Kim ST, *et al.* (2012) Steam-dried ginseng berry fermented with Lactobacillus plantarum controls the increase of blood glucose and body weight in type 2 obese diabetic db/db mice. *J Agric Food Chem* **60**: 5438–45.
64. Kim HY, Kim K. (2012) Regulation of signaling molecules associated with insulin action, insulin secretion and pancreatic beta-cell mass in the hypoglycemic effects of Korean red ginseng in Goto-Kakizaki rats. *J Ethnopharmacol* **142**: 53–8.
65. Lee SH, *et al.* (2012) Korean red ginseng (Panax ginseng) improves insulin sensitivity in high fat fed Sprague-Dawley rats. *Phytother Res* **26**: 142–7.
66. Hong SY, Kim JY, Ahn HY, *et al.* (2012) Panax ginseng extract rich in ginsenoside protopanaxatriol attenuates blood pressure elevation in spontaneously hypertensive rats by affecting the Akt-dependent phosphorylation of endothelial nitric oxide synthase. *J Agric Food Chem* **60**: 3086–91 (2012).
67. Yoo DG, *et al.* (2012) Protective effect of ginseng polysaccharides on influenza viral infection. *PLoS One* **7**: e33678.
68. Ha KC, *et al.* (2012) A placebo-controlled trial of Korean red ginseng extract for preventing influenza-like illness in healthy adults. *BMC Complement Altern Med* **12**: 10.
69. Kim TH, Ku SK, Lee IC, Bae JS. (2012) Anti-inflammatory effects of kaempferol-3-O-sophoroside in human endothelial cells. *Inflamm Res* **61**: 217–24.
70. Paul S, Shin HS, Kang SC. (2012) Inhibition of inflammations and macrophage activation by ginsenoside-Re isolated from Korean ginseng (Panax ginseng C.A. Meyer). *Food Chem Toxicol* **50**: 1354–61.

71. Fan Y, *et al.* (2012) Neuroprotective effects of ginseng pectin through the activation of ERK/MAPK and Akt survival signaling pathways. *Mol Med Report* **5:** 1185–90.
72. Shi S, Shi R, Hashizume K. (2012) American ginseng improves neurocognitive function in senescence-accelerated mice: possible role of the upregulated insulin and choline acetyltransferase gene expression. *Geriatr Gerontol Int* **12:** 123–30.
73. Samukawa K, *et al.* (2012) Red ginseng inhibits scratching behavior associated with atopic dermatitis in experimental animal models. *J Pharmacol Sci* **118:** 391–400.
74. Jung ID, *et al.* (2012) RG-II from Panax ginseng C.A. Meyer suppresses asthmatic reaction. *BMB Rep* **45:** 79–84.
75. Song YB, *et al.* (2012) Lipid metabolic effect of Korean red ginseng extract in mice fed on a high-fat diet. *J Sci Food Agric* **92:** 388–96.
76. Marik PE, Flemmer M. (2012) Do dietary supplements have beneficial health effects in industrialized nations: what is the evidence? *JPEN J Parenter Enteral Nutr* **36:** 159–68.

Conclusion

Medical technology is developing at an astonishing pace. New scientific discoveries raise new hopes in the fight against disease. Governmental and private investments in biomedical research are constantly growing. The biggest investments are currently made in the US, where biomedical research funding increased from $37.1 billion in 1994 to $94.3 billion in 2003; this is doubled when adjusted for inflation.[1] This has facilitated rapidly growing developments in the science of medicine. A large number of new findings are added to MEDLINE (a database that contains publications related to medicine) every year, with nearly 700,000 publications added in 2010 alone.[2] As a result, medical technologies are constantly improving. For comparison, the cost for the sequencing of one DNA nucleotide has shrunk from $10 in 1990, to just one cent in 2005 (a 1,000-fold decrease in 15 years). Even more importantly, new technologies, such as regenerative medicine (stem cell technology), nanomedicine, and pharmacogenomics have been created. These new technologies, along with rapid improvements in existing technologies, continue to advance medical care and have the potential to revolutionize medicine. Below is the summary of the most important possible advances in future medicine:

(1) **Personalization of Treatment** — One of the most noticeable changes in the near future of medical care will be the personalization of treatments using pharmacogenomics (see Chapter 6). The analysis of a patient's genome will be required before a treatment, and doctors will prescribe medicines based on that patient's genetic profile.

(2) **Improvement of Cancer Treatment** — Several major developments promise to improve cancer treatment dramatically. First, as discussed in Chapter 2, new classes of drugs are being developed to fight cancers. This includes antibodies, which will allow treatments to target cancer cells much more specifically than the drugs currently used. Another class is siRNAs, which in combination with some existing drugs, can become a thousand times more powerful in fighting cancer cells. Second, as discussed in Chapter 6, pharmacogenomics will allow the personalization of drug doses for each individual. This will enhance the effect of drugs against different kinds of cancers, and will reduce their toxic effects, two big problems at present. Third, as discussed in Chapter 5, nanotechnology promises to deliver new tools, such as nanotubes, that can specifically find and kill cancer cells. Each of these technologies, taken separately, could dramatically improve cancer treatments. But the combination of them (new efficient drugs, their personalized administration, and nano-tools) might really revolutionize cancer treatment. More cancers should become curable and treatable, with fewer side effects, in the next several years.

(3) **Regeneration of Tissues and Organs** — Several new technologies will contribute to regenerative medicine: stem cell technology, therapeutic cloning, and nanomedicine. Stem cell technology promises to make it possible to replace dead cells and damaged tissues (see Chapter 4). Therapeutic cloning promises to overcome the problem of transplanted tissue and organ rejection (see Chapter 3). Further development of therapeutic cloning may even give the potential to grow new tissue or organs by farming; this process will make the shortage of donor organs a problem of the past. Nanomedicine will facilitate the synthesis of artificial tissues with properties similar to natural ones. It may even make it possible to produce new tissues with advanced properties (see Chapter 5). All of these developments in the field of regenerative medicine could make such common problems such as spinal cord injury, heart failure, Parkinson's disease and others a thing of the past.

How far medicine will go is only limited by two factors: by our desire to develop new technologies, and by our ability to pay for them. Our unwillingness to develop some new technologies is raised by controversies associated with them. However, these controversies are based on moral, ethical, or religious grounds, and those grounds differ depending on country or part of the world. Thus, even if some technologies are prohibited in several countries, they will still develop in others.

Another factor that limits the development of medicine is our resources. Developed countries spend tremendous resources on healthcare. Spending on healthcare in the US alone had hit more than $2.6 trillion in 2011, which was equal to about 18% of the country's Gross Domestic Product (GDP). How much more are we willing to spend? Most developed countries have probably reached their spending limits already. Indeed, analysis has shown that in the US, after a decade of doubling, the rate of increase in biomedical research funding slowed from 2003 to 2007.[3] Nevertheless, developing countries will probably not follow this trend. As developing countries emerge, they will have more money to spend on medical research and development. Therefore, there should be more resources made available in the near future, and the pace of development of medical technologies should also continue to grow.

Governments, and other payers of healthcare costs, are increasingly demanding more quality and value for the amount of money that is spent. One can argue that only those new technologies that significantly improve treatment outcomes should be covered in the marketplace. Thus, it is critical that new technologies be adequately evaluated by sound scientific and clinical studies, so that the relative risks and benefits are well understood before the technology is widely dispersed throughout the marketplace. Society has to measure the value of each new technology against whether or not such technology can contribute significantly to the improvement of health outcomes. Therefore, the field of "new technology assessment" will also assume more and more of an important role in the future.

References

1. Moses H 3rd, Dorsey ER, Matheson DH, Thier SO. (2005) Financial anatomy of biomedical research. *JAMA* **294:** 1333–42.
2. MEDLINE Fact Sheet. (2011) U.S. National Library of Medicine website, Dec 22, 2011.
3. Dorsey ER, *et al.* (2010) Funding of US biomedical research, 2003–2008. *JAMA* **303:** 137–43.

Glossary

Antibody: A protein that serves to recognize and eliminate any foreign substances (antigens) in the body.

Chromosome: The structure of genetic material built from a single double-stranded DNA and associated proteins.

Cloning: Creating an identical copy of something. *Reproductive cloning* is the process of creating a genetically identical copy of an existing organism. *Therapeutic cloning* is the process of creating a body part or organ that genetically matches an existing organism.

DNA (deoxyribonucleic acid): A long polymer molecule that carries genetic information, composed of four kinds of deoxyribose nucleotides (A, T, C, and G).

Epigenetics: The science of genome chemical modifications (such as DNA methylation and protein acetylation), which serve to regulate gene expression without altering the underlying DNA sequence.

Gene: A DNA sequence that encodes an RNA molecule. It is the physical and functional unit of heredity. Previously, a gene was defined as a DNA sequence that encodes a protein molecule. The discussion of the definition of a gene still continues.

Gene expression: The process by which the information in a gene is converted into an observable phenotype. Usually, it includes transcription of a gene into an RNA, and the translation of the RNA into a protein.

Gene therapy: The treatment of diseases by repairing or re-constructing the genetic material.

Genetic engineering: Gene manipulation technology that aims to create organisms with unnatural properties.

Genome: The collection of all the genes from one single cell.

Mitochondrion (pl. mitochondria): A cell organelle that produces energy.

Nanotechnology: The technology that operates with objects, materials, or devices that have one or more critical dimensions between 0.1 and 100 nanometers.

Nucleus (pl. nuclei): A cell organelle that carries genetic information and contains DNA molecules organized into chromosomes.

Non-coding RNAs: A large group of RNA transcripts that do not translate to produce proteins. Micro RNAs (miRNAs) are non-coding RNAs that have a size of 18–25 nucleotides. Small interfering RNAs (siRNAs) are non-coding RNAs that have a size of 20–300 nucleotides. Small RNAs are non-coding RNAs that have a size of 300–10,000 nucleotides.

Pharmacogenomics (Pharmacogenetics): The technology that analyzes how the genetic makeup of an individual affects his/her response to drugs.

Pluripotency: The ability of cells to produce any cell types, except the embryonic type.

Preimplantation Genetic Diagnosis (PGD): The technology that analyzes genetic defects in embryos, before transferring them into the uterus (before implantation).

RNA (ribonucleic acid): A long polymer molecule, composed of ribonucleotides that are created by the transcription of DNA.

Single Nucleotide Polymorphisms (SNPs): DNA sequence variations that occur when a single nucleotide (A, T, C, or G) in the genome sequence is altered. SNPs are an important tool in pharmacogenomics.

Stem cells: Cells that can renew themselves and give rise to specialized cells. *Adult Stem Cells* are stem cells that are found in adult bodies. *Embryonic Stem (ES) Cells* are cells that originate from early (usually five-to-six-day-old) embryos.

Totipotency: The ability of cells to produce any cell types, including the embryonic type.

Vitamin: An organic compound that is required, but cannot be synthesized by, an organism in sufficient quantities.

Index